First published in Great Britain in 2026 by

Policy Press, an imprint of
Bristol University Press
University of Bristol
1–9 Old Park Hill
Bristol
BS2 8BB
UK
t: +44 (0)117 374 6645
e: bup-info@bristol.ac.uk

Details of international sales and distribution partners are available at policy.bristoluniversitypress.co.uk

DOI: 10.51952/9781447378198

British Library Cataloguing in Publication Data
A catalogue record for this book is available from the British Library

ISBN 978-1-4473-7817-4 hardcover
ISBN 978-1-4473-7818-1 ePub
ISBN 978-1-4473-7819-8 ePDF

The author has declared use of generative AI tools in this work. This may include the use of AI for data collection and analysis, language refinement, and/or the preparation of images, figures and tables. Instances of AI-generated or AI-assisted content are identified in the text where appropriate.

Cover design: Bristol University Press
Front cover image: Stocksy/Sibila and Pawel
Bristol University Press and Policy Press use environmentally responsible print partners.
Printed and bound in Great Britain by CPI Group (UK) Ltd, Croydon, CR0 4YY

FSC
www.fsc.org
MIX
Paper | Supporting responsible forestry
FSC® C013604

Bristol University Press' authorised representative in the European Union is:
Easy Access System Europe, Mustamäe tee 50, 10621 Tallinn, Estonia,
Email: gpsr.requests@easproject.com

RISING DEMAND AND DISTRESS IN EMERGENCY CARE

A Sociological Perspective

Daniela Krüger

Contents

List of figures and tables

Figures

Tables

Acknowledgements

I am deeply grateful to all those who supported me throughout this project, from its earliest ideas to its realisation as a dissertation and now as this book, and to all who shared their time and insights along the way.

I would like to express my sincere thanks to Talja Blokland (Humboldt-Universität zu Berlin), whose guidance, encouragement, and belief in my research have been instrumental. I am grateful to have been part of her team and to have benefited from her intellectual generosity and support over the years. Her support of uncommon empirical cases and deep theoretical work as well as her mentorship have profoundly influenced my research. Thank you, Talja!

The department of Urban and Regional Sociology at Humboldt-Universität zu Berlin has been an intellectual home for quite some time and allowed me to exchange and work with many wonderful colleagues and guest scholars. Our department's PhD group was a great place for discussing ideas, issues and express our worries; I always enjoyed reading my PhD colleagues' texts and receive their feedback. Their comments and literature suggestions on an early-stage draft as well as those by my friends were extremely valuable and formed my sensibility for both healthcare professionals and patients as well as their reason-giving. Special thanks go to Nina, Hannah and Robert as well as to Lydia, Jenna and Lina.

To my partner, family, and friends: thank you for your patience, humour, and steadfast support throughout the ups and downs of this process. You are all amazing, and I couldn't have done it without you!

I would like to thank the Heinrich Böll Foundation for generously supporting my dissertation project financially, intellectually, and socially by providing a platform for networks like our research ethics group. I would also like to thank Liane Schenk (Charité – Universitätsmedizin Berlin) for her encouragement and support in her role as my secondary supervisor. I am also very grateful for the opportunity to continue my research in emergency care with wonderful colleagues at the Department of Emergency and Acute Medicine (Charité – Universitätsmedizin Berlin).

I thank Rupert Spurrier at Bristol University Press and Policy Press for his support and guidance through the publication process, as well as the anonymous reviewer for their tremendously helpful feedback on my proposal and manuscript.

Last but certainly not least, I would like to thank my interviewees and the people in the field. I can never thank them enough for the insights they provided into their work and lives. They shared their dilemmas, despair, worries, hopes, laughter, and tears, teaching me thoughtful lessons in the process. I would like to extend my special thanks to the emergency department and EMS gatekeepers. I had memorable interviews with them and their colleagues on the frontlines of these services. I hope this work does justice to the trust they placed in me.

Introduction

> Ms Khan, a student from abroad in her 20s, had been plagued by an enduring flu for some days already, before her sister (a medical doctor living abroad) advised her to see a general practitioner (GP) and get a prescription for medicine. Ms Khan was not fluent in German. She thus searched online for a doctor who is proficient in English. On an online platform, she found a recommendation for an English-speaking GP in a clinic. Coming from a place where GPs work in clinics, too, she 'did not think twice' and ended up going to the emergency department (ED) 'by mistake', she said. (Ms Khan, ED)

> Mrs Dorn was a patient in her 70s. She came with a packed suitcase to the ED and hoped to be hospital-admitted. But when we talked, a patient transport was already ordered for her. 'The doctor says, I'm not an emergency,' she said, disappointed. She described that she had been to the ED more than nine times in the past years, transported by an ambulance – often because she had fallen. Her legs began failing her for years already. She lived alone and had problems providing for herself at home. She wanted to get nursing care but had problems organising it herself. That day she hoped to access nursing care through the hospital admission and the support of hospital staff. (Mrs Dorn, ED)

> Mr Keiser was in his early 30s and came to the ED for a twisted ankle. He did not have a GP as he was 'too young to need doctors [regularly]', he said. Mr Keiser used to come to the same ED with 'small things' before, he explained, as he used to know one of the emergency doctors. He adjusted himself to a longer waiting time in the ED since his acquaintance no longer worked there. Despite the potential wait, he described to prefer the ED over ambulatory care as the waiting for doctoral appointments would take much longer. (Mr Keiser, ED)

Between the sirens and operations of ambulances, between the control for vital signs and admission decisions in emergency departments (EDs), emergency care providers and patients regularly experience mutual disappointment and ambivalence between the urgency of problems and medical help they expect from each other and what they encounter and get. In emergency care, the expectation of frontline workers is that it is *not normal* to call or approach them. According to the *primary narrative* of emergency care, this care provides for the exceptional and rare bodily and psychological extremis (Seim, 2020, p 172): the heart attack, the traffic accident with casualties, the sudden stroke – these cases illustrate that people do not set out to plan such incidents; they often appear to fatefully happen. The rarity of such cases gives the field its temporal rhythm and expectation. Emergency care's public mandate whether in Germany or anywhere else is to be there and be available ('on call') for exceptional needs (Nurok and Henckes, 2009). In order to fulfil their public mandate, the access to emergency care is low-threshold and *open* (Dodier and Camus, 1998, p 414). In an emergency, no appointment is needed, no opening hours need consideration, no insurance status must be proven (Dodier and Camus, 1998, p 414); when a person expresses – or appears to be in need of urgent help, help arrives at any place within minutes and EDs provide their service around the clock and around the year. Emergency care is an extraordinary public service whose low-threshold access has saved many lives since its inception (Montgomery, 1980).

Emergency care's openness is closely related to its *secondary narrative* (Seim, 2020, p 172) for which Ms Khan, Mrs Dorn, and Mr Keiser serve as examples: the field's openness makes the field vulnerable for other uses, potentially undermining its capacity to be there and be available – a fundamental resource dilemma (Lipsky, 2010, p 29). In past decades, patients frequently called 112[1] and approached the ED for mundane, medically low-acute[2] health issues (Ms Khan and Mr Keiser) and for social needs like domestic care problems (Mrs Dorn). While for Ms Khan the access to emergency care appeared so low-threshold she did not immediately notice she was entering an ED and Mr Keiser habitualised going to his neighbourhood ED to wait for less time, other patients like Mrs Dorn stressed the urgency of their request. For many like her, there seemed to be no alternative to calling 112 and going to the ED that day. Emergency care can be a 'safety net' for some (Gordon, 1999; Bourgois et al, 2017).

The low barriers to emergency care gave Ms Khan, Mr Keiser, and Mrs Dorn an initial access to the field, increasing the chances and hopes that the care they expected was awaiting them. With that, the three patients were not alone. Practitioners observed, as one of the emergency medical services (EMS) workers in this book, named Wolfgang, put it, that patients frequently call 112 for symptoms of low medical acuity and hoped for their responsive help. A service for *exceptional needs*, it seemed for many providers in the field, *has become normal* to use, as Wolfgang concluded. Medically low-acute cases appeared to challenge and change the rhythm of exceptionality and rarity of emergency care. From 2018 to 2019, the period during which the fieldwork for this book was conducted, and until today, there has been documented concern about the 'excessive' use of emergency care for low-acuity medical needs and its implications for the provision of emergency care.

Journalists covered the issue in German nationwide newspaper articles with titles[3] such as 'Overcrowded emergency departments: emergency department [as] emergency' (Spiegel, 2018), 'Emergency departments at the limit' (Frankfurter Allgemeine Zeitung, 2018), 'Majority of patients are not emergencies' (Spiegel, 2017) or 'Overloaded fire brigades: "Ultimately, the citizen suffers"' (Gritti, 2018). Similar headlines can be found throughout the research period of this book for the international contexts: 'Emergency Departments under "severe pressure"' (BBC, 2018), 'Emergency departments overwhelmed by patients, not meeting targets' (New Zealand Herald, 2018), 'Why the emergency room is always crowded and what we can do about it' (Friedman and Pauly, 2020). The headlines of such articles indicate a central but implicit aspect of the debate: the *excessive* and *false* use of emergency care is not only a functional issue but also a moral one (Moskop et al, 2009). After all, patients' *wrong* choices can, in its worst case, endanger other people's well-being or their lives.

Practitioners and researchers expressed their concern about phenomena termed 'crowding' (in EDs) (Morley et al, 2018) and 'overuse' (of ambulances) (see Kawakami et al, 2007), describing them as a potential risk to patient safety. 'Crowding' and 'overuse', that is, the exhaustive use of emergency care services, are assumed to be associated with prolonged waiting times for patients for ambulances and ED treatments, which could affect patients' treatment outcome and health (Searle et al, 2015; Lowthian, Cameron et al, 2011; Lindner and Woitok, 2021). In this context, researchers sought to understand patients' 'misuse' and 'inappropriate' use of emergency care services to plan for interventions (Murphy, 1998; Dejean et al, 2016). In Germany, healthcare insurance companies and medical associations commissioned expert reports on developments and potential reasons for the presentation of so-called 'non-emergencies' (see, for example, Kassenärztliche Vereinigung Berlin, 2017). In such reports and further studies, authors classified a share of patients as low-acute, not requiring emergency care from a perspective of medical urgency (see Sefrin et al, 2015; Günther et al, 2017; Mangiapane et al, 2021).

Internationally, estimations about medically low-acute cases range between 30 per cent and 40 per cent of all cases in EDs (Carret et al, 2009; Uscher-Pines et al, 2013; Wahlster et al, 2020; Slagman et al, 2023) and up to 30–50 per cent in the EMS (Sefrin et al, 2015; Lowthian, Cameron et al, 2011; Schubert et al, 2022). While scholarly work from the 1970s suggests that low-acute patients in the field are not a novel observation (see Roth, 1972;

Schwartz, 1975), their specific increase along with a general increase of patients appeared to be a more recent development (Lowthian, Cameron et al, 2011; Berchet, 2015; Scherer et al, 2017, p 645; Schubert et al, 2022).

The average annual growth rate in Germany for ED visits between 2005 and 2011 was about 5 per cent, whereby the growth rate of countries in the Organisation for Economic Co-operation and Development (OECD) was about 2 per cent (Berchet, 2015, p 10).[4] This is consistent with the 5 per cent average annual growth rate in the German EMS between 1994 and 2013 (Sieber et al, 2020), which amounted to a 50 per cent total increase between 2005 and 2015[5] (Seeger, 2019, p 7). Despite a drop during the COVID-19 pandemic, the annual growth rate of ED utilisation continued in Germany (Statistisches Bundesamt [Destatis], 2024), and other contexts (see, for example, Lopes et al, 2023). Although it remained unclear to what extent low-acuity patients were responsible for this trend and the apparent rise in demand in Germany, they had nonetheless been at the centre of debate and a major source of concern among providers.

Patients with issues of low-acuity appeared to strongly mismatch the mandate, professional expertise, capacities, and expectations in emergency care, demonstrated by providers' and researchers' descriptions of patients' 'inappropriate' utilisation or 'misuse' of their services (Murphy, 1998; Carret et al, 2009; Hudgins and Rising, 2016). Despite increased and constantly high numbers of patients and their in part 'inappropriate' use of services, policy makers, managers, and planners in hospitals and the EMS kept the access to the field open – that is, they have refrained from strictly regulating who may access the ED or call EMS and receive hospital transport, despite suggestions in policy debates to, for example, introduce a monetary fee to deter low-acuity patients from visiting the ED (Deutsches Ärzteblatt, 2018). What were the consequences for professionals and low-acute, mismatching patients?

This book is about cases like Ms Khan, Mr Keiser, and Mrs Dorn.[6] It studies the ways in which low-acute patients' use of healthcare, planners' and managers' institutional access regulation and health service providers' gatekeeping of healthcare-related services mutually influence their access to (symbolic) resources (for example, legitimacy of urgency, recognition as professional, healthcare-related services and information). More specifically, it is about how patients and providers negotiate legitimacy of urgency and a sense of professionalism in the field, and how patients with medically low-acute (and social) needs appeared to collectively take the field *out of sync* of serving the bodily and psychological exceptions – and thus changed providers' expected *normal* conduct in the field. It was a change that planners and managers did not initially put a stop to institutionally, and which 'looped back' (see Barnard, 2019) into the field and its intricate social arrangements.

Figure 0.1: Ambivalence of emergency care

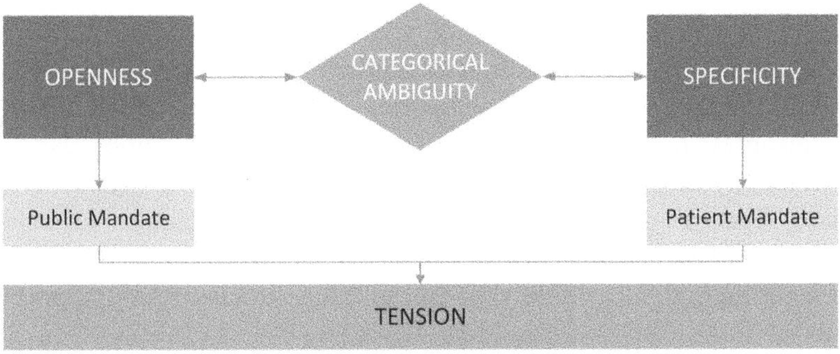

Source: Based on the conceptual work of Dodier and Camus (1998)

Despite the openness of the field, emergency care is also very specific (Dodier and Camus, 1998): the field has a specific institutional arrangement, mandate, training, and funding, focused on on-call, brief and intense medical care to save lives. The specificity of emergency care may thus not meet the individual medical and/or social needs that low-acute patients carry into the field; in a sense, undermining the field's openness (see Figure 0.1; Dodier and Camus, 1998).

With this increase in mind, and considering that a share of people with low-acuity problems call 112 and pass through the ED, this project asks: what happens to these patients as they carry a problem they deem urgent into (para)medical[7] encounters with professionals whose mandate it is to rescue people's lives? Healthcare workers are part of the 'good professions' with caring ideals (see Fassin, 2008; Hillman, 2016). Does this logic benefit patients also when they mismatch the classification of life rescue in the field? Or, in contrast, do they get rejected or discriminated against as they appear to use the service 'falsely' and 'inappropriately' or even appear to 'misuse' it (potentially to the detriment of other, high-acuity patients)?

In turn, what happens to professionals who experience challenges to their vocation and changes to their work as seemingly more and more patients of low medical acuity call 112 or present to EDs? How does an assumed rise in low-acute patients influence their work, (symbolic) resource access and the relation to patients – but also to their superiors? Planners and managers of health services are caught in the middle between being responsive to their frontline workers as co-workers and patients as their mandator. Therefore, the book asks: how did planners and managers respond to rising patient demand, part of which was understood to consist of low-acuity cases? With what consequences for the field's institutional arrangement, and frontline workers' and patients' relations and resource accesses? In short: what happens in a social field, when a classificatory practice appears to change? What are the associated symbolic gains and losses for the three main actors in the field, both collectively and individually?

The aim of the book is twofold. Empirically, it aims to explore the ambivalence arising from the 'openness' and 'specificity' of emergency care (Dodier and Camus, 1998) and its differential consequences for the access to resources for different social agents and their relations among each other. Conceptually, it aims to show how the relatedness of social agents in a field mutually influences their (symbolic) resource access. The book explores consequences for people working in emergency care (providers; frontline workers),[8] people planning and managing the field (planners, managers, superiors), and for patients with low-acute complaints who attempt to access services in the field. To address the book's aims, it draws on ethnographic fieldwork in the EMS and several EDs in *Urgencity.*[9]

Urgencity is a pseudonym for a large German city, in which the study was conducted. Providers in *Urgencity*, as well as in other cities around the world, saw an increase in the number of patients seeking emergency care (Schwartz, 1975; Lowthian, Cameron et al, 2011; Lara-Millán, 2014; Berchet, 2015; Scherer et al, 2017; Andrew et al, 2020; Sieber et al, 2020). Methodologically, I conducted over 300 hours of participant observation in three EDs and at four EMS stations in *Urgencity*. In addition, I carried out 34 interviews with a total of 42 planners, managers, and providers, as well as 66 patients. To further contextualise and validate the fieldwork, I also participated in conferences and expert forums on emergency medicine and its changes and challenges.

The data were used to map the field and its struggles, and ultimately to study the drivers and consequences of the increased – and constantly high number of patients for agents in different social positions, their access to resources, and their relationships with each other.

Research on the increasing demand and distress in emergency care

So why do low-acute patients call 112 or present directly to the ED? In general, utilisation researchers find three clusters of 'patient motives' (Schmiedhofer et al, 2016) for low-acuity 112 calls or emergency department visits in Germany and beyond: first, patients come or call because they 'don't know any better' (Ms Khan); second, because patients 'use it strategically' (Mr Keiser); and third, because patients 'can't help it' (Ms Dorn). Specifically, the researchers identified factors such as health anxiety, desire for time autonomy, unfamiliarity with healthcare systems, desire for access to a medically highly equipped environment, barriers to timely appointments with outpatient physicians, as well as low health literacy and (psycho)social needs (see Luiz, 2008; Luiz et al, 2002; Searle et al, 2015; Scherer et al, 2017; Schmiedhofer et al, 2017; Redelsteiner, 2018; Somasundaram et al, 2018; Breuer et al, 2020; Ruegenberg et al, 2024). For approximately two decades, the study of patients' reasons for low-acuity ED visits and EMS calls has been a prominent area of health services research (Kraaijvanger et al, 2016; Coster et al, 2017; Vogel et al, 2019). And while these findings offer valuable insights, they often share a common limitation in adopting a discipline-specific approach that focuses on individual-level motives, also known as 'methodological individualism' (Emirbayer, 1997). While I agree that patients' individual reasons are both empirically as well as analytically relevant, especially in encounters where providers scrutinise them for legitimacy, we still know little about their sociological underpinnings.

Beyond individual motives for calling 112 or presenting to the ED, there is another critical question: what are the outcomes and consequences of the rising demand and mismatch of some patients in emergency care settings? Research has focused on patient safety, waiting times, and satisfaction with care (Hoot and Aronsky, 2008; Johnson and Winkelman, 2011; Morley et al, 2018). While patient safety, that is, the prevention of harm to patients (Institute of Medicine Committee on Data Standards for Patient Safety, 2004, p 35), and waiting times are tied to the self-interest of a patient and thus a relevant research domain, it leaves other stones unturned. It leaves open the question of patients' self-rated outcomes of their care in the ED or the EMS. Although satisfaction has been measured and typically scores high, it remains a somewhat opaque construct (Williams et al, 1998). It tells us little about how patients navigate care settings in detail, what matters to them and why, or how do they respond in encounters in which the legitimacy of their request may be questioned.

Turning to the provider perspective, existing literature has shown that labour disputes over ED and EMS working conditions and pay are associated with increased workloads (see Jacobs et al, 2013; Jacobsson et al, 2020; Seim, 2020). While these findings are also important, we do not gain an understanding of the impact of rising and constantly high patient numbers – especially in regard to the low-acute patients – and discrepancies on providers' self-understanding, and daily work and encounters with those patients. In contrast, emergency care managers and planners remain notably absent from most empirical work. The research that does exist is almost always limited to discussion papers and reactions to policy proposals (see, for example, Augurzky et al, 2018; Sefrin, 2024).

Overall, what remains underexplored is how these dynamics unfold relationally – between patients, providers, superiors, and planners – and how they express and reshape expectations around emergency care access, and result in symbolic losses and profits. As Veenstra and Burnett (2014, p 189) suggest, addressing these dynamics requires moving beyond substantialist ontologies that treat motives and outcomes as isolated, self-contained attributes. To that end, this book adopts a sociological lens grounded in

Bourdieu's field theory (esp. Bourdieu, 1977, 1990; Bourdieu and Wacquant, 1992), and his understanding of fields as sites of *classificatory struggles*.

Emergency care is a good case to study classificatory struggles: the general increase in the number of patients and the relevant proportion of patients with low acuity has led to public and internal struggles over who should legitimately have access to emergency care (for what needs and why), or how emergency care is organised (how open or specific its access should be), and why there is an increased use of services at all. In practice, struggles are evident on multiple empirical levels: when individual patients negotiate with providers for recognition of their perceived need or urgency; when providers struggle for professional recognition with patients and their superiors; and when planners, working on the future of emergency care organisation, find themselves somewhere in the middle and caught between the need to be responsive to their frontline colleagues and to patients with their needs.

To understand both the social and collective drivers behind low-acuity calls or presentations, as well as its consequences for patients and professionals alike, this book employs a theoretical framework that guides the analysis and contributes to the broader literature on the topic.

The theoretical framework: relatedness, embodiment and feel

The book's framework is based on and builds upon the social theory of the French sociologist Pierre Bourdieu. The framework consists of intricate, interconnected concepts that describe and explain social life and action, with field, habitus, and capital serving as its core elements (see Bourdieu, 1990; Bourdieu and Wacquant, 1992). His theoretical approach is not an unusual choice. In fact, it has become increasingly popular among researchers studying health and healthcare-related topics. As Collyer (2018; also Veenstra and Burnett, 2014) points out, authors have particularly applied certain concepts such as habitus and capital to analyse health practices and behaviours, and their relation to health outcomes. However, these authors did not always address the interconnectedness of these and other concepts. As Collyer (2018) notes, a key concept of the Bourdieusian approach has been notably absent: the concept of the *field*. Without this concept, researchers would often conceptualise healthcare systems as 'containers' within which social action takes place (Collyer, 2018, p 116), or as structures that straightforwardly determine individuals' choices and behaviours (Veenstra and Burnett, 2014, p 191).

Studying healthcare as a field – that is, as composed of differently positioned and equipped agents who struggle in 'direct' and 'indirect' exchanges over, for example, the provision and utilisation of healthcare and thus access to resources – enables a relational, multi-level, and multi-actor analysis of emergency care (see Bourdieu, 2018a; Shim, 2010, p 6).[10] It offers a perspective to resolve the duality between a healthcare structure vis-à-vis agents and practices within it, and to understand the functioning of the healthcare system in relation to their histories, social hierarchies, and socially unequally distributed capacities to influence its structure and conduct at the institutional and everyday level (Shim, 2010; Collyer, 2018).

The analysis presented in this book is guided by Bourdieu's understanding of the concept of field as a 'field of struggles' (Bourdieu, 2018a, p 136). In an abstract sense, Bourdieu assumes that every social field consists of a hierarchical social space[11] in which individuals quietly negotiate or overtly struggle with unequal means to maintain or subvert classifications of meaning and value (Bourdieu, 2018a, p 6). Most often, these struggles are about naming things, actions, and people, and consequently granting or denying access to field-specific resources (Bourdieu, 2018a, p 6) – processes that often go unnoticed and appear *natural*. With that in mind, the constant high demand for emergency care, along with the daily negotiations in EDs and the EMS regarding waiting times, diagnostics, and admission decisions reveal a more fundamental issue than just conflicts over a service. Patients, providers, and planners become differently positioned and equipped social agents in a struggle over historically grown professional and lay positions, and mutual recognition for their needs and status. To gain a better understanding of the social mechanisms underlying such classificatory struggles, their drivers, and consequences, the three concepts of *relatedness*, *embodiment*, and *feel* are derived and the latter expanded from a Bourdieusian perspective.

The exploration of the conceptual triad begins with *relatedness*. This concept can be understood as a defining analytical and empirical characteristic of a field. It provides insight into why and how struggles and change unfold within social fields. Thus, relatedness serves as the meta-concept from which *embodiment* and *feel* are derived (see Figure 0.2).

Although *embodiment* and *feel* are two sides of the same coin, they differ in conceptual orientation, as envisioned by Bourdieu (1990, p 67). *Embodiment* refers to the pre-reflexive inscription of fields into the body and their reproduction through perception and practice (Bourdieu, 1990, pp 54–6). *Feel* denotes the practical expression of embodiment to seemingly effortlessly navigate the field (see Bourdieu, 1990, p 67). As an anticipation sense (Bourdieu, 1990, p 66), it also responds to, or is exposed by rupture or change within the field – and, in line with relatedness as an integral characteristic of fields, loops back into and shapes the field itself.

This book emphasises both concepts to illuminate how a specific contextual change and the struggles surrounding it – the processes commonly described in the literature as *deprofessionalisation* – unfolds within the field of healthcare, and how such change feeds back into its complex web of social relations, positions, and shared understandings among patients and professionals in emergency care. Understanding deprofessionalisation is essential for grasping

Figure 0.2: Relation between core concepts

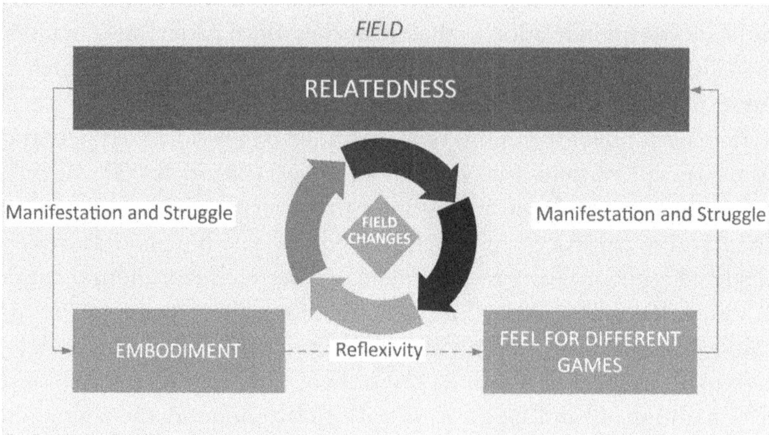

both the field's interrelatedness with other fields and the dynamics of emergency care, as well as the observations analysed in this book. Accordingly, the concepts are first discussed theoretically and then related to empirical observations of healthcare transformation in the existing literature.

Relatedness of everyone and everything

Relatedness is the key characteristic of a field. Put simply, a field in Bourdieusian understanding is a 'bundle of relations' in which everything and everyone is related (Bourdieu and Wacquant, 1992, p 16).[12] This notion of relatedness underpins how positions and relations, as well as power and legitimacy between and within fields are structured and contested. In this book, relatedness refers to three central aspects:

First, an agent's position in the field becomes meaningful only in relation to others (Silva, 2016, p 171). Positions and their objective relations take the forms of for example, domination, subordination, homology (Bourdieu and Wacquant, 1992, p 97). For instance, an agent's dominant position is related to – and requires – the domination of others. Conversely, this means that an agent's changing field position also affects others in that field. Thus, a change in a field position shakes up a complex arrangement of positions, relations, ways of being, and value distributions in a field (Veenstra and Burnett, 2014, p 189). The later discussed shift in the position of healthcare professionals in relation to patients, and vice versa, will serve to illustrate this.

Second, field positions are not randomly assigned; they are backed up by '[a] species of power (or capital)' (Bourdieu and Wacquant, 1992, p 97). Power is expressed and accumulated through capitals – in other words – through the ability to define and (de)value those capitals (Bourdieu and Wacquant, 1992).

Symbolic profits and losses are therefore understood in this book as the (de)valuation and (un)recognition of capitals that agents consider or attempt to mark as (un)valuable, whether in everyday encounters or in institutional terms (see Bourdieu, 2011). Bourdieu differentiated between three fundamental forms of capital: 'economic' (for example, assets, money), 'social' (for example, social relations and profitable networks), and 'cultural' (for example, knowledge, skill, and certified trainings).[13] A person's specific capital endowment, along with the particular capital structure – that is, the types of capital that matter within a given field – determines their position in that field. For these capitals to be effective, they must be recognised as legitimate. This is where *symbolic capital* comes into play. Bourdieu (1990) conceives of symbolic capital as a form of legitimacy. It is the 'recognition of authority as legitimate' by misrecognising the involvement of power (Loveman, 2005, p 1655).

Such forms of capital are not easily acquired; they embed and reflect historical struggles within a field and accrue over time, granting access to various forms of profit and shaping the objective relations and positions among agents (Bourdieu, 1990, 2011). In professional fields such as healthcare, expert knowledge serves as symbolic capital layered onto cultural capital (Schinkel and Noordegraaf, 2011, pp 85–6),[14] exemplifying this dynamic: it is both a 'stake' and a 'weapon' in social struggles (Emirbayer and Johnson, 2008, p 11). Those who historically lack it can be kept at a distance (Bourdieu, 2018b, p 106) because they lack the necessary 'professional acclaim' (Schinkel and Noordegraaf, 2011, p 89). Those who have it are drawn closer to the field (Bourdieu, 2018b, p 106). And those agents who possess field-specific capital in greater amounts than others are drawn closer to the power centre of the field (Hage, 2011), which means they can impact its structure and the conduct of the field. Bourdieu thus likens field-specific value or capital to 'trump cards', which can gain or lose relative value within a field depending on its dynamics and ongoing struggles (Bourdieu and Wacquant, 1992, p 98).[15,16]

Third, fields are only semi-autonomous (Emirbayer and Johnson, 2008, p 3). Because they are embedded within and connected to other fields, they must continually defend their specific logic against both internal and external pressures. Particularly in pluralist societies, the dynamics, struggles, and likelihood of field change are heightened (Bourdieu and Wacquant, 1992, p 102; Silva, 2016). A field's *doxa* is its core logic; it remains dominant only as long as it is not significantly challenged by powerful external fields or by *heterodox* agents – those who hold views that oppose the prevailing doxa (Bourdieu and Wacquant, 1992, p 101). In other words, everything rises or falls in a field with the status of its doxa – that is, what individuals embodied as valuable (capital), including specific objects, practices, themselves, and others, as well as how they orient their actions and reflections (habitus and feel) (see Bourdieu, 1990; Bourdieu and Wacquant, 1992). Agents, therefore, connect a part of their whole being to a specific field doxa (Bourdieu, 1990). As such, struggles and changes within a field and the related symbolic losses can be deeply unsettling for some agents; challenging them, quite literally, to the bone.

Analytically, as Emirbayer and Johnson (2008, p 22) observe, field struggles occur both vertically and horizontally: horizontal struggles arise between fields, while vertical struggles occur within them. In healthcare, horizontal struggles are reflected in ongoing debates about deprofessionalisation. From this perspective, external fields and their logics such as corporate management, legal regulation, and bureaucratic accountability are said to have increasingly shaped the practice of healthcare and resulted in professional contestation (Timmermans and Kolker, 2004; Betz and O'Connell, 2014; Timmermans and Oh, 2010). Deprofessionalisation is also linked to vertical struggles, such as those between providers and patients as collective agents. Timmermans (2020) argues that the contemporary patient differs from the passive recipient of care typical of the 20th century. Today's patients are more actively involved in managing their health and in medical encounters than ever before, increasingly questioning and even challenging the professional hierarchy (Timmermans, 2020, p 266).

Embodiment of the past

In this book, embodiment refers to the historically shaped collective and individual capabilities (capitals) and expectations of providers and patients within the field of emergency care (see Bourdieu, 1990). Agents' equipment with these are shaped by their respective positions within the field and are inscribed into agents' dispositions[17] as ways of perceiving, thinking, and acting – what Bourdieu describes as *habitus* (Bourdieu, 1990; Bourdieu and Wacquant, 1992).[18] The habitus thus 'ensure[s] … the active presence of past experiences, which, deposited in each organism in the form of schemes of perception, thought and action, tend to guarantee the "correctness" of practices and their constancy over time, more reliably than all formal rules and explicit norms' (Bourdieu, 1990, p 54). Habitus, therefore, encompasses both 'internalization' – what shapes the individual – and 'externalization' – how the individual, in turn, shapes the field (Wacquant, 2016, p 65).[19]

In relation to agents' capital-based social positions and dispositions, which manifest in their expectations, this book uses the term 'position-taking' to describe expressed expectations and other forms of articulated dispositions (see Emirbayer and Johnson, 2008). Position-taking, thus, literally relates to the taking of positions in a field, that is, 'semiotically' or 'culturally' signifying actions, statements and so on (Emirbayer and Johnson, 2008, p 26). Taking a position, symbolically locates agents vis-à-vis others (for example, superiors, peers, patients), either in distance or proximity. In other words, position-takings as expression of habitus may be understood as relational work (see Lamont and Molnár, 2002).[20]

Further, I use habitus as embodiment to explain the historical commonalities and differences between and within healthcare providers and patients as well as their different capacities to provide, navigate, or negotiate within healthcare settings (see Bourdieu and Wacquant, 1992). Within healthcare itself, different professions share commonalities. For example, nurses and EMS workers share dispositions that are part of the 'medical habitus' of doctors which is connected to scientific biomedicine, technical competence, and skill (Nettleton et al, 2008; Brosnan, 2009; Johannessen, 2018b), while also showing specific dispositions which separate them from the medical habitus. Nurses' habitus focuses stronger on care and cure (Carter, 2014); paramedics' habitus has a stronger focus on brief medical intervention and transport to rescue (Nurok and Henckes, 2009). The habitus is an expression and (re)producer of commonalities of a field as well as the specific field position of occupational sub-groups. As fields are nested, we can zoom in and find subfields with their own and shared logics, rules, and regularities (Bourdieu and Wacquant, 1992, p 104). We can also zoom out and find a subfields-encompassing field with, to a certain degree, a shared logic, rules, and regularities – although it entails 'a genuine qualitative leap' between the field levels as Bourdieu and Wacquant (1992, p 104) write.

The 'qualitative leap' (Bourdieu and Wacquant, 1992, p 104) between healthcare providers and patients is considerable, rooted in the expert–lay divide and the corresponding differences in capital endowment. This divide has historical origins in the professionalisation of healthcare. When the medical profession emerged, the state[21] granted it exclusive jurisdiction over healthcare and manifested the powerful status of this profession vis-à-vis others with symbolic capital (Hupe, 2012; Timmermans and Oh, 2010, p S95) – thus with a 'field-specific form of status' (Schinkel and Noordegraaf, 2011, p 79). Here, the relatedness of positions in fields is evident. 'Professionalism, … is a scarce resource' and is based on exclusive rights to claims, occupational and social closure, and on the implicit recognition of the claim to do so as legitimate (Schinkel and Noordegraaf, 2011, p 87). Scientific biomedical knowledge, expertise, and skill – institutionalised and monopolised in trainings, curricula, and certification (cultural capital)[22] and developed by professional associations (social capital) – has formed the corner stone of healthcare professionals' powerful position (symbolic capital) (Luzio, 2006; Schinkel and Noordegraaf, 2011; Hupe, 2012, p 40). Professions defined socially relevant problems and monopolised the means and knowledge necessary to solve them (Luzio, 2006, p 550).

Monopolisation, in turn, created relations of dependency and positions of power and subordination. Professionals became experts whose power was based on their exclusive embodied knowledge and practised skill; patients became laypeople marginal to the field, lacking expert knowledge, and dependent on professionals and their problem-solving capacities (Luzio, 2006;

Lorenzen and Zifonun, 2012). While patients became historically dependent on providers due to the lay–expert divide; professionals, too, are dependent on those they serve. Professions must assert a commitment to the public good in order to maintain public legitimacy (Luzio, 2006; Timmermans and Oh, 2010; Hupe, 2012). This claim and its recognition matter both for the profession as a whole and for its individual members. The powerful social position of professions and the public trust in their conduct are mutually reinforcing (Luzio, 2006, p 556). Luzio (2006, p 556) writes:

> A belief that the profession is grounded in moral values must … be present if the client is to rely on members of the profession to maintain high standards. We trust that standards derived from the ideals of a universalistic orientation, of economic disinterest and of service to the good of the public welfare will be kept.

Similar to providers, patients share habitual commonalities as well as differences. Regarding commonalities, sociologist Merton (1976, p 71) reflects on the etymology of the term patient in his 1976 publication, noting that patients were historically understood as 'calmly expectant, quietly awaiting the course of events'. Patients assumed the 'sick role' (Parsons, 1991 [1951]) seeking medical care when unwell in order to regain health with their habitualised provider; they largely accepted the dominance of the medical profession by following doctoral advice and treatment (Timmermans, 2020, p 261; Stivers and McCabe, 2021), and trusting in the monistic service ethic of the medical profession (Luzio, 2006). Concerning habitual differences, researchers pointed out that patients are socially differently equipped to navigate healthcare systems and their settings as well as negotiate with healthcare providers (Shim, 2010; Willis et al, 2016). Shim (2010) uses the term 'cultural health capital' (CHC), while Willis et al (2016) refer to 'system knowledge' to describe healthcare-specific forms of skill, knowledge, and experience that enable individuals to engage effectively with providers and the healthcare system as a whole.

The habitus concept allows to conceptualise collectivity, unity, and cohesiveness within social groups. Habitus may also be used to describe fragmentation, tension, or friction (Silva, 2016; Wacquant, 2016).[23]

As noted earlier, everything rises or falls in a field with its doxa. The tendencies of deprofessionalisation are likely to challenge the habitus of both providers and patients. Scholars describe how professional work under austerity regularly limits frontline workers' practice (Clayton et al, 2015). Also, shifts from public service work to managed for profit work (McDonough, 2006; McDonough and Polzer, 2012) or from tacit and embodied knowledge to standardised protocols and their audits (Nettleton et al, 2008) bring about conflicting new logics to which professional agents' habitus may be temporarily ill adapted. Bourdieu termed the temporal ill adaptation or lag of the habitus as *hysteresis* (McDonough, 2006, p 635). Hysteresis is a condition in which 'dispositions function out of phase and practices are objectively ill-adapted to the present conditions because they are objectively adjusted to conditions that no longer obtain' (Bourdieu 1990, p 62). The loss of *illusio* (*disillusio*) is related to hysteresis. When losing illusio, agents break with the immanent sense of the field, so that it appears 'absurd' and 'future-less' (Bourdieu 1990, p 82). The result may be disengagement from a field (Nurok and Henckes, 2009; Clayton et al, 2015).

Horizontal and vertical field struggles have given rise to assumptions about deprofessionalisation. These developments have also left their mark on the habitus of patients. In the latter half of the 20th century, there was a notable increase in public suspicion of medical autonomy, accompanied by a concurrent erosion of the rationale justifying the monopoly of medical practice and knowledge (Timmermans and Oh, 2010; Timmermans, 2020). Timmermans (2020) suggests this period as the foundation for the emergence of the 'engaged patient'.[24] According to this, today's patient is not only more responsible for their own health but also has greater access to information and knowledge about it. The dramatic increase in access to health-related and healthcare information is discussed as another key development in the transformation of collective positions and relations between patients and providers (see Nettleton and Burrows, 2003).

The information asymmetry between healthcare providers and patients, which constituted part of the professional monopoly, decreased as a result of the growing availability of information and knowledge from patient advocacy groups and online resources, providing alternative sources of medical information to that of the doctor (Stivers and Timmermans, 2020; Stevenson et al, 2021). Furthermore, the accessibility of diagnostic devices challenges not only the monopoly that doctors have traditionally held over diagnostic means but also the interpretation of those diagnostic results (Lupton and Jutel, 2015). The advent of diagnostic apps and devices offering at least some diagnostic interpretation may represent a further challenge to the traditional role of doctors in the field (see Lupton and Jutel, 2015).

It is Timmermans' (2020) contribution that the evolution of the engaged patient is not only based on the increase of knowledge (the 'expert patient') or on the market forces creating a 'patient as consumer', but that it takes different, mostly congruent transformations together and assumes their effects on the shift from an authoritative patient–doctor relationship to more cooperative forms (Stivers and Timmermans, 2020, p 62). In light of the challenges to medical legitimacy and hegemony, patients were compelled to alter their evaluation of the individual medical encounter and the healthcare profession (see Stivers and Timmermans, 2020; Timmermans, 2020). This shift in perspective involved a reconsideration of the traditional patient–provider relationship and the assumption of unquestioned trust. Instead, it is argued that patients began to assume the potential influence of previously non-medical ethics and logics that potentially guide medical practice. The monistic ethical framework constituted the basis of impersonal trust, which may subsequently be negatively affected (Timmermans and Oh, 2010). As the field changes and the agents' embodied conception of their social world evolved, the nature of the medical encounter itself also underwent transformations.

Feel for different games

Bourdieu, like other sociologists, used the mundane analogy of 'games' to help explain his theoretical approach (for an overview: DiCicco-Bloom and Gibson, 2010). For Bourdieu, 'games' refer to 'field' (Bourdieu, 1990), the disparate terms are indicative of differing conceptual emphases, which have been less acknowledged in sociological literature. With his conceptual differentiation, Bourdieu refers to agents' level of awareness for the dynamics in a field and capacity of agents to employ purposeful action (McDonough, 2006, p 634). Instead of being *in* the field of healthcare and naturalising it as a matter of fact – the doxic effect of power in a field – the field dynamics are seen, questioned and, potentially, critiqued – a state that Bourdieu (2018a, p 72) described as *allodoxia*. The conceptual notion of field, in other terms, describes how 'agents do not apprehend the constitutive role of their beliefs and actions … and, hence, misrecognize [the field] as an external, naturally given reality' (McDonough, 2006, p 634). In this regard, agents fail to comprehend the field in its organisational and social hierarchal context. Conversely, Bourdieu (1990, p 66) established the 'feel for the game' as a complementary concept to the field and habitus, in which agents demonstrate a certain degree of awareness. To be *in* the game signifies that agents can 'play' it and thus are able to make deliberate attempts to influence the outcome (Bourdieu and Wacquant, 1992, p 99).

Bourdieu's conceptual differentiation is thus useful in describing the social mechanism behind the shift in the patient's engaged position in healthcare. The level of awareness of being *in* the game allows for purposeful, directed action (Veenstra and Burnett, 2014, p 189). In the era of patient engagement, the doxic effect of the medical profession may have diminished. However, this does not imply that patients possess comprehensive knowledge about their healthcare provision, and social inequalities exert a considerable influence. In this regard, Bourdieu's notion of 'feel for the game' differs importantly from rational conceptions of strategising agents who are assumed to have full knowledge of a situation (Veenstra and Burnett, 2014, pp 190–2). Instead, in Bourdieu's understanding, insight is limited and depends on agents' field-specific capacities or their field-specific capital to understand and work the field (Bourdieu, 1990, p 63).

I understand patients' feel for games as a sense for determining a symbolic loss or profit, that is, whether a provider acknowledges a patient's urgency and assumable has the patient's best interest in mind – or rejects patients' needs for assumable illegitimate reasons ('playing another game' of, for example, time efficiency, profit, unresponsive standard routine). The feel determines the assumed (il)legitimacy of a provider's practice and relates to the notion of trust. I suggest to understand trust, in Bourdieusian terms, as the illusio of a field or the 'commitment to the presuppositions – doxa – of the game' (Bourdieu, 1990, p 66). Implicitly, this shows that patients, too, embody in their habitus certain expectations of providers and healthcare. These expectations can be broken.

For the book two notions of trust and distrust are important: 'institutional' or 'public (dis)trust' in social institutions such as biomedicine, the healthcare system, the medical profession and 'impersonal (dis)trust' in a provider based on their association with a profession (Misztal, 1996; Luzio, 2006). According to Luzio (2006, pp 557–8), it is in the encounter where patients meet providers face to face as 'representatives of the profession' that impersonal trust in the profession can be negatively affected or positively reaffirmed. Institutional (dis)trust can manifest as (dis)illusio and (dis)engagement from the doxa that healthcare is 'best' organised by the medical profession. Impersonal (dis)trust may be understood as (dis)illusio of the doxa that professions commit themselves to the public good and have the patient's best interest in mind. Departing from this, the encounter can also be the site where patients come to perceive that a provider is not a good representative of the profession, while trust in the profession itself remains unaffected (see Luzio, 2006).

As patients and professionals take different positions *in* the field, they take different positions *on* the field or game – thus their 'feel for the game' differs.[25] Today's patients exhibit distinct practices that require a specific skill set. The advent of the engaged patient thus brings the concept of 'capitals' back into focus. In reference to Bourdieu, Shim (2010) has coined the concept of 'cultural health capital' (CHC) to further conceptualise a specific form of capital that patients embody, encompassing skills, competencies, and styles valued by providers in healthcare. CHC builds on Bourdieu's habitus, and thus is part of the patients' embodied repertoire of skills and know-how. Shim (2010, p 11) writes that 'CHC – following Bourdieu's notion of habitus – is mobilised in largely unconscious, habitual schemes of perception, thought, and action that are embodied through experience and socialization and deeply stratified.' CHC can thus be conceptualised as the embodied skill set of patients, while the *feel* represents the sense that builds on it and is actively mobilised, for example, when patients and providers meet face-to-face in a medical encounter.

Shim's (2010) CHC is important in showing how social inequalities operate and are reproduced in an encounter by focusing on the provider's judgement.

However, because it follows the provider's evaluation of the patient's actions or resources as valuable or not, it remains analytically unidirectional. While the significance of this concept and its value for examining the reproduction of social inequalities in medical settings cannot be overstated, it is not sufficient in considering how patients utilise CHC to assess the effectiveness of their care and the provider who delivered it. The 'feel for the game' or its extension as 'the feel for different games' now turns the focus on the patient and their assessment of what they consider 'right' or 'wrong' when encountering a provider, placing heightened attention on cues with regard to providers' assumed intentions and potential breaches in ethical standards that have accompanied the rise of patient engagement. This evaluation is based on patients' varying levels of CHC and the premise that they either extend or withhold trust during or in an encounter, rather than automatically trusting by default (Luzio, 2006, p 557).

It is assumed that patients engage their 'feel for different games' for three reasons: first, the interaction between patients and providers remains characterised by a competence gap and informational asymmetry, which renders the control of providers' actions an impossibility (Luzio, 2006, p 552). Second, trust in a provider may be considered a 'risky investment', given that the provider is not personally known (Luhmann, 1979, p 24 in Luzio, 2006, p 553). In an epistemological context, in which patients assume responsibility for calculating risks and making informed choices regarding the 'right' care (see Timmermans, 2020), this risk may even appear of greater weight. Third, the shift in responsibility for patients' health and a growing awareness of the changing logic of healthcare provision (for example, commodification) may result in a lack of automated trust. Patients may feel the need to determine which 'game' a provider is playing, as patients may assume breaches of the monistic ethic.

Similar to patients, providers also develop and mobilise a feel for patients' games – but for other reasons. First, medical practice is characterised by uncertainty in terms of medical conduct (Holmes and Ponte, 2011). In recent years, scholars suggest different accountabilities have added uncertainty to the medical practice (Timmermans and Oh, 2010; Hupe, 2012; Seim, 2020). Professionals, in other words, do not categorically practice in autonomy by drawing on their professional authority; professions get organised (see Freidson, 2001; Calnan, 2015). As such, providers face multiple accountabilities to patients, professional peers, supervisors, the accounting and management structures of their home organisation, and other organisations with which they cooperate (Hupe and Hill, 2007; Seim, 2020). Intersections with these different social fields and their 'pulls' (Hage, 2011) demand providers to situationally prioritise different social, professional, market, or bureaucratic values (Nurok and Henckes, 2009). The *feel* is thus a relational operator. It weighs the prioritisation of different – often conflicting – logics over that of others.[26]

Second, the shifting position of the patient as engaged left a collective trace on providers. Scholars show how providers use their 'sixth sense' or embodied professional knowledge and experience to vet patients' expressed needs and urgencies in emergency care for authenticity (Johannessen, 2018a; Wamsiedel, 2020). Strategising to a certain degree, secrecy and even lying in provider–patients relations is not a new social phenomenon (Fainzang, 2002). But as Timmermans (2020, p 269) writes '[o]ver the past decades, patients have started to talk differently in physicians' offices. Less intimidated by white coats, they have become more assertive, even if they tend to eschew open conflict.' Part of providers' feel is to anticipate this new challenge and decide how to respond to it (un)responsively.[27]

The following section outlines the methodological approach that guided the study and shaped how this framework was translated.

Mapping the field through relational methodology

Using Bourdieu's field approach required applying a relational methodology, which in turn demanded determining the boundaries of the field under study. As fields are often intertwined, overlapping, and spanning, empirical research must set analytical boundaries, while remaining cautious not to reify the object of study. Many interview- and observation-based studies focus on a specific social group, place, or organisation (Desmond, 2014, p 547). While such studies may adopt relational methodologies, they risk intentionally or not reifying bounded entities and social classifications (McQuarrie and Marwell, 2009, p 253; Desmond, 2014). As Desmond (2014, p 563) notes, this may lead to neglecting relations across groups and sites.

To counter this, Desmond (2014) proposes a 'relational ethnography', which 'involves studying fields rather than places, boundaries rather than bounded groups, processes rather than processed people, and cultural conflict rather than group culture' (Desmond, 2014, p 574). Following the recommendation of Collyer (2018, pp 121–2), I first focused on the horizontal struggles among powerful institutional agents to understand field-defining discourses and tensions. In 2017, I started applying for field access, making first explorative interviews with ED managers, followed by several providers, and planners (see Appendix for a detailed method report). These first interviews combined with attendance of events and policy document research allowed me to map a wider field to explore and identify 'core actors' (see Desmond, 2014, p 570): the EMS, EDs, and patients (see Table 0.1). In a vertical perspective, I related differently positioned agents in an organisation, namely: superiors (that is, planners, managers), providers at the service frontline, and patients. Using the notion of the *chain of rescue*, I understand my field as crossing different organisations and hierarchies; this occurred to me as a reasonable step as, first, the EMS's and EDs' cooperation is

Table 0.1: Relational dimensions of study

	Agents and positions
Horizontal relations	EMS
	EDs
	Patients
Vertical relations	Superiors, planners
	Providers
	Patients of different social position

institutionalised (Ahnefeld, 2003), and, second, interviewees named struggles between and within organisations as relevant to their service provision.

Sampling different cases and different hierarchies or positions within a case allowed the study of the mutual (un)making of boundaries between and within fields or organisations; it allowed studying conflict and cooperation and what may be constitutive of them (see Hammersley and Atkinson, 2010, p 28).

In order to provide a deeper understanding of the healthcare context in which this research is situated, the following section offers an overview of the institutional structure of the German healthcare system and its key institutions. Particular attention is given to the historical struggles that have shaped the current system and their implications for both patients and providers. This background helps to illuminate the institutionally embedded expectations that providers bring into their encounters with patients, and it illustrates the structural position and responsibilities patients hold within the system. Where appropriate, comparisons will be drawn to other healthcare systems to contextualise the German case and enable clearer analytical positioning.

Emergency care provision within a 'double structure'

Germany's healthcare system is a corporatist model in which the medical profession and Statutory Health Insurance (SHI) funds coordinate healthcare (Kuhlmann et al, 2009, p 515). SHIs cover most of the population (Kuhlmann et al, 2009, p 515). A smaller share of the population (8,7 million, around 10 per cent) is insured in Private Health Insurances (PHI) (Statista, 2020).[28] While healthcare planning in other countries is state-central (for example, Great Britain), in Germany corporatist bodies negotiate healthcare provision and planning with the state (see Döring and Paul, 2010; also Busse and Blümel, 2014). The federal state provides the legal framework and monitors compliance with it; the self-administration is responsible for the detailed organisation (Busse and Blümel, 2014, p 55). The federal state delegates responsibility to plan and provide healthcare to the physicians' associations,

SHI funds, and hospitals (Döring and Paul, 2010, p 535; Kuhlmann et al, 2009, p 512). Thus, self-governing corporatist bodies have a significant influence on the form and content of German healthcare.

The Federal Committee[29] represents the central self-governance board in German healthcare (Busse et al, 2017). Physician and hospital associations as well as SHI funds and their votes lead the Federal Committee (Busse et al, 2017, p 884). Other social agents (for example, patients, other healthcare sub-professions such as nurses, paramedics) are marginal to the board and to healthcare planning (Kuhlmann et al, 2009, p 515). This arrangement results from historical struggles for professional autonomy and standing between associations, and professionals and patients.

Only since 2004, the Federal Committee has included patient representatives and the German Hospital Society as members (Kuhlmann et al, 2009, p 515). Even though the former have only advisory and not voting rights (see Federal Committee, 2022), Kuhlmann et al (2009, p 520) see the inclusion of patient representatives as an extension of patients' 'active participation' in German healthcare planning, which at least to some extent reflects their changing social position.

Struggles in the 19th century centred on office-based doctors and sickness funds (Busse and Blümel, 2014, p 26). Reflecting the sectoral divide in German healthcare, later struggles involved the medical profession itself. In the 19th century (and until very recently), most doctors practised office-based and developed associations of powerful standing (Busse and Blümel, 2014, p 26). Hospitals used to focus on nursing care before they began to provide curative care and employ medical doctors (Sefrin, 2003, p 624). Hospital doctors and office-based doctors and their associations began to compete for ambulatory patients, that is, those patients who leave a practice after treatment (also called 'outpatient care') (Gerlinger, 2017).

Ambulatory doctors lobbied for their exclusive responsibility over outpatient care and curative measures (Busse and Blümel, 2014, p 28); their exclusive responsibility marginalised other non-doctoral professions like nurses, midwives, and communal services and largely prevented hospital-based doctors from practising outpatient care (Busse and Blümel, 2014, p 28). The state granted office-based doctors the monopoly over ambulatory care in 1931 (Busse and Blümel, 2014, p 28); a decision that Busse and Blümel (2014, p 28) describe as a 'major collective victory for office-based physicians over sickness funds, hospital-based physicians, medical officers in community health and other health care professionals'. The SHI Physicians Act in 1955 confirmed the division (Gerst, 2015; Leber and Wasem, 2016, p 3).

The struggles within the medical profession and among associations furnished healthcare as provided in two separate sectors, that is, in hospitals and ambulatory practices (Luzio, 2004, p 427). The two sectors are 'organized differently along the lines of planning, financing, organization and governance' (Blümel et al, 2020, p xxv). Whereas federal states plan and invest in hospital care and organise the EMS, physicians' associations administer and organise outpatient care in self-organised practices (Luzio, 2004, p 426). Ambulatory doctors organise in regional associations.

Every federal state has a regional SHI physician's association that organises ambulatory outpatient care locally for SHI patients. These associations and their doctors enter a 'service guarantee contract' with the federal state and sickness funds (Döring and Paul, 2010, p 536). Compared to other European healthcare systems, the German model, in which doctors provide specialist medical care on the basis of often self-employed doctors in individual or joint practices, is rare (Gerlinger, 2017). Most medical specialists in other healthcare contexts are hospital-employed or practise in larger care units (Gerlinger, 2017).

The provision of emergency care mirrors the German 'double structure' of specialist medical care (see Gerlinger 2021, p 10). Providers organise acute care in both sectors, separated by the degree of symptom severity: the EMS and hospital EDs are responsible for acute and life-threatening situations that (are likely to) result in stationary inpatient care; ambulatory doctors (that is, general practitioners and specialists) are responsible for acute and less severe health problems within practice opening hours and as out-of-hours service (Blümel et al, 2020, p 162) (see Figure 0.3).

In detail, the Regional Associations of SHI Physicians have organised an out-of-hours care hotline (116 117) since 2012 and out-of-hours care in on-duty practices and by individual (and changing) on-duty ambulatory doctors (Blümel et al, 2020, p 162). Hospitals provide emergency care on a 24/7 basis in EDs. Patients may approach an ED by self-referral, doctoral (ambulatory) referral, or be transported by an ambulance (following a 112 call). At the ED, the ambulance crew presents the patient to a nurse or a doctor (Blümel et al, 2020, p 166). Medical doctors of different specialisation (for example, surgery, internal medicine) and nurses work together in an ED, which is managed by a chief doctor. In some cases, ED managers employ paramedics and rescue workers – initially trained within the EMS system – who then work alongside nursing staff. Hospital-based emergency care is delivered by both for-profit and non-profit hospitals. This stands in contrast to the EMS, which is provided exclusively by non-profit organisations (Blümel et al, 2020, p 166).

Fire brigades often in cooperation with aid organisations[30] arrange and provide the EMS at the level of the federal states and on a 24/7 basis (Blümel et al, 2020, p 163). Each fire brigade includes a control centre, where dispatchers process 112 emergency calls. Across Germany, there are around 250 such control centres. When a 112 call is received, a dispatcher usually assisted by a dispatch software determines whether to send an ambulance staffed by a rescue worker, paramedic, or an emergency care doctor, depending

Figure 0.3: Patient pathways in German acute and emergency care

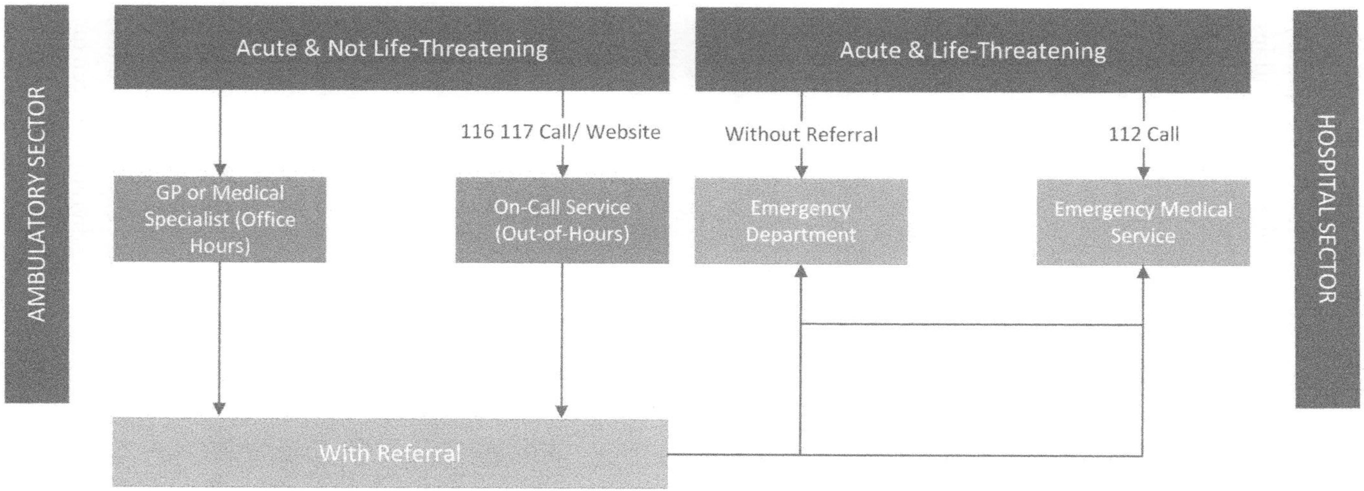

Sources: Based on Blümel et al (2020, p 166) and SVR Gesundheit (2018)

on the assessed level of medical urgency (Blümel et al, 2020, p 163). Predefined arrival times vary by federal state (Blümel et al, 2020, p 163).

Two types of emergency vehicles are primarily in use: ambulances and emergency physician vehicles (Blümel et al, 2020, p 164). An ambulance is typically staffed by two personnel whose qualifications may differ. An emergency physician vehicle is generally staffed by a paramedic and a medical doctor (Blümel et al, 2020, p 164), reflecting the higher-severity calls that these teams respond to. Depending on the case severity, staffing may include paramedics, rescue assistants, or rescue paramedics, the latter holding the lowest level of paramedical training (Blümel et al, 2020, p 164). Since the implementation of the Emergency Paramedics Act in 2013 in Germany, the training for rescue assistants has been phased out and replaced by the more advanced paramedic qualification (Blümel et al, 2020, p 164). The financing of EDs and EMS follows a dual structure, consisting of reimbursement through statutory and private health insurance (SHI and PHI) and, in some cases, out-of-pocket payments (Blümel et al, 2020, p 164). Additional funding is provided by the federal states (Blümel et al, 2020, p 164).

Between medical providers, patients have free choice of doctors. Germany is, institutionally speaking, a non-gatekeeper system (Reibling and Wendt, 2012). If a person experiences an acute health problem, they have multiple options to get medical help. They may approach an on-duty ambulatory doctor in an ambulatory practice,[31] call the emergency hotline of the ambulatory on-call service (116 117) for advice and, for example, a home visit, or self-assess their symptoms online (https://www.116117.de/de/patienten-navi.php). Different to other healthcare systems which employ gatekeeping, in Germany, patients may directly go to a hospital ED (without a doctoral referral) or call 112 for immediate help and hospital transport. In countries like Denmark or Great Britain, patients may consult with their General Practitioner (GP) or emergency hotline staff first, to then decide on further medical help (Seeger, 2019, p 40). In Denmark, specifically, patients cannot self-refer to an ED without medical referral (Seeger, 2019, p 40).

Germany has many healthcare facilities and providers and few access regulations. *Freie Arztwahl* – the free choice of doctors – suggests choice and autonomy for patients. In practice, such choice may also be experienced as challenging. For example, rather than having one unified emergency hotline, Germany has two that concern health issues (112 for the EMS and fire brigade, and 116 117 for on-duty ambulatory care; similar to other countries like Spain, UK, Finland, Denmark), reflecting the system's sectoral division; whereas other countries without strong division between the sectors organise out-of-hours urgent care units on a walk-in basis (for example, UK), the division of sectors still complicates this in Germany (Seeger, 2019, p 40). Urgent and emergency care offered by ambulatory doctors, the EMS, and EDs appears for many as difficult to navigate (Blümel et al, 2020, p 165).

The services, as Blümel et al (2020, p 165) write, 'work often in parallel and are not well connected'.

Health service researchers assume that the open and fragmented arrangement of emergency care in Germany contributes to the patient increases that EDs and the EMS observe (Seeger, 2019; Blümel et al, 2020, p 165). At least in part, as this overview demonstrated, this may be based on the 'organisation-centeredness' (Redelsteiner, 2018), division, and struggles between ambulatory and hospital care. Such an arrangement relies on the functionally right choices of healthcare 'consumers' (see Kuhlmann et al, 2009), and may stipulate emergency care providers' gatekeeping and moral evaluation of such choices.

The book will lay out how navigating healthcare has a normative dimension, and the evaluation whether people use healthcare 'rightly', to rephrase Timmermans and Epstein (2010, p 70), is a more or less 'subtle' way to enforce a powerful institutional arrangement and reproduce its 'normality'.

Overview over the book

The book is divided in three parts.[32] Part I lays the empirical groundwork for the forthcoming Parts II and III. It outlines the core principles and classifications of the field, the expectation of regularity and the struggles between work hierarchies in emergency care provision concerning the definition of 'the emergency'. It demonstrates the value and ambiguity of the emergency category in practice, which creates difficulties for – and tensions between – planners and frontline workers. Furthermore, Part I presents providers' 'social diagnoses' for the increase in emergency care, offering broad insights into providers' observations of changes in *Urgencity* and in emergency care. These observations position providers within the field in relation to their superiors, peers and patients by referring to the relational work they undertake when presenting reasons for observed changes. These positions of providers will be reflected in the following parts, where the book focuses on encounters with patients and the consequences of changes in emergency care.

Part II shows that accessing emergency care is neither linear and straightforward for low-acute patients, nor is providing emergency care to low-acute patients for providers. The part zooms in on encounters between providers and patients along the chain of rescue, examining how low-acute patients navigate healthcare settings and engage with providers. Ultimately, it shows how both patients and providers negotiate access to resources. In doing so, it addresses patients' attempts to make providers responsive to their needs, how providers vet patients' needs for legitimacy and patients reflect on their ED visit and its outcome. The 'chain of rescue', which encompasses the first aid measures from EMS care to ED care, serves as analytical trajectory, following two logics: synchronous or single encounters between a patient and a provider, and diachronous trajectories of multiple encounters between one patient and several providers. This approach allows, first, to study the complexity of negotiations and gatekeeping at different individual moments within the chain of rescue. Second, it allows to study the relational 'work' that patients do along their trajectory of several encounters with providers.

The final part of the empirical analyses rounds off the current developments in *Urgencity* by describing the consequences and resulting dilemmas faced by planners and providers due to the rising demand in the field. Part III begins by looking at the dilemmas faced by providers as they regularly encounter patients with (psycho)social needs that cannot be accommodated in their work. It then addresses how these dilemmas travel to those who plan and make decisions, driving formal classificatory change and adding to the underlying dilemmas for superiors and planners: being more responsive to patients with mismatching needs and acknowledging a broader definition of 'urgency' means being unresponsive to providers and their position on a narrower definition of 'the emergency'. In other words, consolidating low-threshold access to emergency care for mismatching patients had unintended consequences, resulting in some providers' *hysteresis* and *disillusion*, with some leaving the field.

Looking at the symbolic side of rising demand in emergency care allowed this book to address the fact that there is more to an encounter with an EMS crew for patients than receiving a transport; it also showed that there is more to an encounter with a low-acute patient for frontline workers than providing a health service. Many patients hoped to receive reassurance, support, and legitimacy in a complex and often unresponsive healthcare system, while many providers sought professional value and recognition in their work, hoping to fulfil the task of saving lives and maintaining a public mandate, despite the field's conflicting resource dilemma. Low-threshold emergency care and its high demand complicated the access to recognition for both patients and their providers. The concluding chapter of the book reiterates the original research interest of the book and points out its main empirical and conceptual findings in context of the debate on deprofessionalisation. It will also provide a discussion on the limits and benefits of the working with Bourdieu's field approach and concludes the chapter with suggestions for future research and policy implications of the empirical findings.

PART I

Classifying 'the emergency': moral economies and social diagnoses of change in emergency care

Chapter 1 lays out the core beliefs of emergency care that carry and (re)produce value. Emergency care is organised as an on-call service. Policy and decision makers have planned emergency care to provide care for exceptional – life-threatening or risky – illnesses and injuries (see Ellebrecht, 2020). Such emergencies are rare, and the field and frontline workers are equipped and trained to respond to them (Jeffery, 1979; Palmer, 1983; Nurok and Henckes, 2009). The rarity and exceptionality of emergencies then give the field its specific moral economy and high social value, influence quantity in equipment and staffing, require focused training and protocols, and lead to shared habitual expectations of those working in the field. In other words, fields function, as Hansen et al (2014) suggest, as moral economies in which, following this analogy, agents engage in symbolic and moral struggles over values or the 'right' and 'best' classifications and practices.

Chapter 1 shows that categorising 'the emergency' and deciding on the care for medically low-acute patients is not straightforward and instead involves classificatory struggles along work hierarchies, especially between providers at the service frontline and their superiors who share and differ in their habitual commonalities.

Chapter 2 zooms out of the focus on emergency care to give frontline workers 'social diagnoses' (Brown et al, 2011) of the increase and constantly high patient numbers. These diagnoses are insightful narrative markers on what providers consider 'normal' or 'right' to situate themselves vis-à-vis patients, communities, superiors, and other health services providing agencies, and lays the ground for the impact of field changes on providers' expectations and professional self-understanding.

1

Beliefs in unambiguous categories and institutional arrangements

Chapter 1 marks the beginning of the empirical section of the book and delves into three critical aspects of emergency care. First, it explores how institutional frameworks not only set out the paths and tasks within emergency care but also embody moral economies. These frameworks perpetuate entrenched beliefs about the 'right' and 'wrong' ways to seek medical help, shaping and sometimes clashing with the socio-cultural expectations of what constitutes an emergency. Low-acute patients regularly challenge these doxic beliefs, in Bourdieusian terms, revealing the ambiguities in emergency categorisation.[1] Second, the chapter draws on Pierre Bourdieu's concept of habitus to discuss how professionals internalise and perpetuate the field's logics and values through expectations – integrating the objectified history of their profession, such as mandates, standards, and social positions. This sedimentation of professional logics shapes the moral economy of the field, reinforcing a collective belief system and validating the field's operational logics. Third, there is a nuanced examination of how both providers and their superiors recognise the necessity of broad definition and access to emergency care to ensure no emergency is overlooked. However, this expansive definition of what constitutes an emergency introduces ambiguity. This leads to differing standpoints between frontline staff and superiors on how to handle low-acute patients.

Dividing up the field: two jurisdictions and 'one problem'

Even if the arrangement of a healthcare system appears natural or given, scholars argue that they are the result of historical and on-going struggles within and among professions and other agents (for example, policy actors, patient representatives) (Collyer, 2018, p 122; Tilly 1998, p 181). This section introduces into the struggle between the ambulatory and hospital care agencies in providing emergency care in *Urgencity*.

Despite the marginal position of patients in planning the healthcare field's setup (see Introduction), the position of patients is reversed in the question of who must initially define the emergency. The field depends on patients (or third parties) and their 'right' categorisation of symptoms. Each minute lost in determining an emergency can endanger patients, but if they (or others) call 112 and go to an emergency department (ED), instead of an ambulatory doctor, for an issue of low medical acuity, they bind resources to the 'wrong places', possibly endangering others and increasing workloads and costs. The reliance on patients' self-assessment and the low-threshold access to the ED has produced tension between the local Contracted Physicians' Association (CPA) and hospital EDs in *Urgencity*. The original mandate for ambulatory emergencies lies in the jurisdiction of local CPAs. Many ambulatory patients were, however, treated and examined in EDs, as Dr Weber laid out:

> By [German] law, section 75 Social Code V, the responsibility for ambulatory emergencies rests solely with contracted physicians. We are actually not allowed – we do it of course. … if someone comes to see us, we connect this to a mandate of action. … the key sentence is: 'The patient votes with the feet.' That means that he [sic] comes to us because he himself [sic] or a third party defines him [sic] as emergency.

Dr Weber's description encapsulates the struggle between the sectors. There are separate jurisdictions for ambulatory and hospital emergencies that regulate reimbursement (section 75 Social Code V). At the same time, there is a lack of a clear definition to separate the ambulatory emergency from its hospital counterpart (Seeger, 2019, p 20).

Hospital emergency care developed from primary care, further distancing and specialising as a sub-profession by claiming jurisdiction over symptoms which occur in a particular time frame (within hours) and express a particular severity (life-threatening) (Timmons and Nairn, 2015, p 9). To ensure safety and low-threshold access to services, emergency care laws and policies do not qualify 'the emergency' with specific biomedical indicators. Instead, patients or third parties initially self-assess and determine the need for emergency care. Dr Weber and others referred to definitions of a German emergency care association (DGINA) as well as the local emergency medical services (EMS) law. The DGINA is a German non-governmental organisation (NGO) advocating for the interests of emergency medicine and its providers in Germany.

An emergency or emergency patient for the DGINA is 'any person who exhibits physical or mental changes in health for which the patient or a third party deems immediate medical and nursing care necessary' (Behringer et al, 2013, pp 625–6). Local EMS laws define emergencies as a person being in 'life-threatening conditions' or 'who are likely to suffer serious damage to their health if they do not receive immediate and appropriate medical help'.[2] The guidelines of the DGINA and the local EMS acts guarantee a low-threshold access to potentially life-saving care; they also give room for ambiguity.

Dr Lindemann explains:

> So, medical emergency, there is a nice definition from our medical society, this is defined by the patient, right?! And if there is someone

> with a panic attack or is very unhappy or is having constipation for three weeks or something like that, those are all people [who think]: 'No one comes to help you', and I also help them gladly, but I know that from the [point of] disease severity it's ambulatory level.

The field's definitions produce openness and low-threshold access, on which life-rescue depends (Dodier and Camus, 1998, p 414); at the same time, it gives the right and the initial classificatory responsibility to patients (or third parties). People expect categorisation can be used to 'solve organizational problems', yet the use of categories often creates new problems (Tilly, 1998, p 11). The ambiguous category of 'the emergency' serves as example. The doxic division between sectors obscures historical, intra-professional struggles as well as the development of expert knowledge on health and healthcare and its unequal distribution; professionals and lay-people alike are left with the belief that naturally there are 'right' and 'wrong' ways of getting medical help and that the orientation and sorting into 'right' medical settings is based on unambiguous definitions and clear boundaries that laypeople and practitioners can follow (see Timmons and Nairn, 2015). From the providers' perspective, these expectations also inform the choice to enter the profession.

Central 'tools of the craft' of emergency care

Public service habitus: 'helping people, serving society'

Why do people become doctors, paramedics, nurses, and fire fighters – in short, professionals in helping others? While Desmond (2006, 2007) showed how the general habitus of working-class 'country boys' equipped wildland fire fighters with the disposition to be 'naturally' good at their work, this section shows that providers internalise ideas, skill and expectations about emergency care as part of the field's illusio early on in life as well; it can explain why people 'gravitate' (Hage, 2011) towards certain professions. The stakes of a field inform expectations of what the field is about. The expectations stay with providers during their years of practice (see also Maynard-Moody and Musheno, 2003, p 12). The expectations concern the social and professional value of their work, that is, to whom and which purpose they serve – expectation in 'what to be good at' and 'why to be good at it'. Although rescue workers, paramedics, ED nurses and doctors differ in their social positions, training, and field positions,[3] I argue that they share commonalities in their dispositions, as *helpers* who serve a *common good*. The field's stake and profession's value justified the burdensome and risky work (see Desmond, 2007).

The development of a specific habitus does not begin when entering a professional field as organisational member. People develop and cultivate their habitus over the course of their lives (Staab and Vogel, 2014).

Bourdieu uses the concept of a 'trajectory' to illustrate this process (Staab and Vogel, 2014). The trajectory constitutes the exposure to the various fields that agents encounter 'synchronously' (at the same time) and 'diachronously' (over their lifespan) (Silva, 2016, p 170). The habitus can thus be termed 'embodied history', functioning as the memory card of these exposures (Bourdieu, 1990, p 56). In other words, the habitus captures and shows the traces of agents' positions, capital endowment, engagement and exposure to multiple fields and is just as nested as fields are intertwined and overlap (Bourdieu, 1990).

The power of professions lies in the largely unquestioned recognition of their legitimacy and social value that translates between fields (see Bourdieu, 2018a, p 125). People are socialised, early on and throughout life into the symbolic value and cultural categories of teachers, police officers, fire fighters, nurses, and doctors. Related expectations and the value of certain professions circulate widely and exert a draw on some people, often corresponding with social classifications, such as gender, class, race and ethnicity (see Desmond, 2006; Desmond, 2007; also Watkins-Hayes, 2009). Dispositions of the primary habitus do not determine social trajectories, but they increase the likelihood for occupying certain social positions such as specific occupations (Staab and Vogel, 2014, p 164; Wacquant, 2016). Many providers whom I asked about their interest in joining the EMS or fire brigade, the nursing or medical field described their orientation of 'helping others' and 'serving the common good'.

Anton who was a group leader within an EMS station, had studied and worked for years in the private sector. His description represents that of many others I encountered in the field. He described ways into and reasons for joining the field.[4] Anton said that his way into the fire brigade was 'very random'. After years in his job, he 'started questioning' what he was doing and had 'problems to respect his own role in society'. ' [Y]ou start questioning yourself at some point: "Why am I doing this? And what is my actual motivation?"' He had friends in the fire brigade that thought of him as a 'good match' for it and the EMS; after an internship that convinced him to join the fire brigade, he started his new job and training. Anton described what he referred to as 'idealism' and the desire to help others that mattered for him and many of his co-workers when considering to enter the service:

> The notion of helping which is of course very very inflationary used to and certainly can be interpreted in many many ways. But yet most have some motive that guides them into such a specific and exhausting job. Well, but basically in the background there is always the thought 'to serve society a service' and 'to help out people who are in distress in any way'.

Helping and having the mandate to help drew many into entering their current positions as doctors, nurses, fire fighters, and EMS workers. Such a motivation may not be understood as an individual driver but as a collective driver, energy, or force (Wacquant, 2016). While the habitus varies in time and space and across power, there are commonalities, and there is a certain coherence across domains of practice, such as social classes, lifestyles, or professions, as Wacquant (2016, p 66) argues. Next to helping the individual patient in need, providers also expressed an orientation towards their public responsibility.

McDonough and Polzer (2012, p 359) described the development of the 'public service habitus' by people working in state services. As an orientation towards the public good, the public service habitus is an expression (and reproduction) of a historical public mandate. Many providers in the fire brigade and EMS are civil servants,[5] while providers in the hospitals are employees of communal, private, or charitable hospitals. Despite the shift and diversification of hospital ownerships, frontline workers expressed position-takings that stressed their public task. Dr Meinhard said that they were following a public service mandate (*Versorgungsauftrag*). Dr Weber similarly explained they had 'the legal mandate for emergency care for the citizens of [*Urgencity*]'. Providers in the fire brigade and EMS stressed their embodiment or mediation of the state (see Douglass and Calnan, 2016, p 397); some said they embodied ('we are the state') or are an emblem of the state ('we represent the state').

To serve the public, staff in EDs and the EMS had to translate, sort, and hierarchise needs and urgencies of individual patients. The next section addresses a standard, the triage, which supported practices of categorising and sorting.

Triage: categorising urgency, sorting patients

Triaging is the central tool of their trade, as nurse Tim explained to me on my first day of observation. EDs and the EMS are people-processing settings (Schwartz, 1975; Lipsky, 2010). Triaging sorts patients according to medical urgency and structures the workflow in emergency care. Other public service provision contexts also use triaging to organise their workflow. It can generally be understood as '[a] model for differentiation among clients in people processing [contexts]' (Lipsky, 2010, p 106). Categorising people aims at optimising the use of resources when patient numbers exceed resource capacities (Lipsky, 2010, p 106). For emergency care, sorting and prioritising treatment reverses the problem of a high patient demand. It allows selection of high-acuity cases from low-acuity cases and a prioritisation and focus of resources (see Ellebrecht, 2009, pp 231–2). In a context of high patient numbers, sorting is of vital relevance.

The EMS triages patients and their cases as well. The 112 dispatcher uses a medical priority dispatch system for a first assessment, leading to alarm keywords and priority categories.[6] At site, EMS workers collect vital signs of patients as part of a first assessment; they note the impression of the patients' medical urgency on a protocol that they exchange with the staff in the ED. In the ED, an additional triage determines the time that can pass until a patient needs to be seen by a doctor, according to triage guidelines.

When patients enter the ED, no matter if 'by foot' (without private transport or EMS) or transported by the EMS, patients are triaged by a triage nurse (that is, a nurse who underwent training in conducting these assessments), less often by a triage doctor. Two medical dimensions are relevant to triaging: measuring the objectifiable symptoms of the body, called vital signs (for example, body temperature, blood pressure, heart rate), and asking patients for the intensity of the pain they feel (in case the patient is responsive). The Manchester Triage (MTS) became a widely applied standard that many professionals, hospitals, and EMS use. The standard consists of five categories, identified by colour, that indicate degrees of medical urgency (Christ et al, 2010). These triage colours are synonymous for patients' medical urgency.

In the ED, the provider who conducts the triage writes a protocol and clips it to a coloured folder, which informs doctors and indicates the time frames in which the patient should be seen: red[7] equates to life-threatening conditions that need immediate consultation (0 minutes to be seen by a doctor); orange means 'very urgent' and equates to 10 minutes; yellow means 'urgent' and equates to 30 minutes; green means 'standard' and equates to 90 minutes; and blue means 'non-urgent' and equates to 120 minutes of waiting (Gräff et al, 2014).[8] In the ED, nurses check on patients in intervals and reassess their conditions and possible changes that indicate a changing degree of medical urgency. Many studies verified triage systems before they became standard algorithms in medical settings (see Christ et al, 2010). Their aim is to reliably identify the most urgent among many cases (Christ et al, 2010, p 892) to increase patient safety and quality of emergency treatment despite moments of high workload.

Triaging helps the field sustain its logic of being on high alert, and supports professionals in their quest to help. The MTS, like other standards in the field, sustains the doxic focus on the vitality of the body. Guidelines for emergency care lay out schemes and Standard Operating Procedures (SOPs) to identify and handle medically urgent situations: guidance for reanimation, specific SOPs for respiratory, circulatory problems, strokes or trauma, that is, heavy injuries, and so on. Standards are homologous to the doxic understanding of the functionally right medical paths and the disposition of the helpers that help when 'the world of patients lies in pieces', as Anton referred to medical emergencies. Standards such as the triage reproduce the field's focus on the acute and severe problems of the body.

Medical standards tame, as Holmes and Ponte (2011, p 164) pointed out, a sense of medical uncertainty, and they make, as Lipsky (2010, p 59; 122) wrote, people and their complex social circumstances appear 'manageable', a core task of bureaucratic logic. The triage offers objectifiable benchmarks to order medical urgency seemingly unambiguously. Classifying is, however, as the next section shows, not a straightforward task. Despite the existence of standards such as the triage, agents in the field struggled over defining what an emergency entails.

Classifying the emergency

The difference between 'being' and 'experiencing' an emergency

Barman (2013, p 104) writes, '[c]lassification systems … entail the symbolic demarcation of phenomena into the discrete categories of social life'. A problem with classifying the emergency is the drawing of clear categorical boundaries to specify which clinical symptoms and markers the category entails a priori, and which not (Timmons and Nairn, 2015, p 6). Despite its ambiguity, many frontline workers suggested an exclusive set of symptoms and situations when they described the emergency.

EMS worker Wolfgang said an emergency is when a person is wearing their 'head under the arm', a metaphor for severe injury or physical trauma. Henrik added, 'leg off', 'person run over by train', 'fallen from house', and infarcts. Others classified stroke, cardiac arrest, panic attacks, loss of consciousness, or breathing difficulties as emergencies. To classify what an emergency is, providers also specified what it is not: using labels such as 'bullshit', '*Pillepalle*' or '*Bagatelle*' (both describe trivias), and 'garbage'. Instead, 'real', 'classic', 'actual', and 'medical', to were related to emergencies. These designations come close to what Steensland (2006, p 1273) described as cultural category, that is, as notions that reinforce 'the symbolic and programmatic boundaries between categories'. Even if the emergency appears as a 'continuum' of symptoms and situations (Seim, 2020, p 26; 58), as 'biological pathology' and 'social phenomenon' (Timmons and Nairn, 2015, p 6), the cultural category facilitates the creation of unambiguity by suggesting a coherent clinical definition and narrow boundaries between 'false' and 'right' or 'inappropriate' and 'appropriate' use, while there is no such clear definition (see Murphy, 1998).

Patients and providers often had different views on the urgency of a problem. Providers differentiated between 'being' or 'experiencing' an emergency (see Table 1.1). Many talked about people 'being an emergency' as a state that they intersubjectively evaluated and confirmed as legitimate. Medical emergencies like strokes or heavy injuries fit objectifiable clinical parameters and SOPs. In contrast, 'experiencing' an emergency is something patients 'feel personally' (EMS provider Anton), is 'subjective' (ED nurse Evelyn), and 'depends on the perspective' (ED nurse Catherine), possibly mismatching a 'real' emergency.

Table 1.1: Service frontline differentiation of emergencies

Emergency determined as:	Objectifiable	Subjective	
Emergency classified by:	Patients, third parties, frontline workers	Patients	
Emergency labelled as:	Real emergencies	Experienced emergencies; misuse	
Emergency request is:	Legitimate, authentic, common sense	Legitimate, authentic, common sense	Illegitimate, inauthentic, against common sense

'Real' emergencies ranked high in the field, but providers did not automatically dismiss 'subjectively felt' emergencies as illegitimate cases; they distinguished between different forms of *helplessness*. Like station manager Mr Leidner, many differentiated a 'justified' and 'unjustified' need for help. Mr Leidner elaborated this distinction, when answering my question if there is a boundary between justified and unjustified reasons to call 112:

> So, I say it's *der gesunde Menschenverstand* [the common sense] … Every one of us, even if he [sic] gets [somewhere] the 4th time that night, is overtired and in a bad mood, when he [sic] realizes that for the one who called there was very probably a situation that he [sic] could not handle, where he [sic] was [uncertain] … where he [sic] was unsure. So, the definition for him was really life-threatening, for the one he [sic] called for or for himself, then he [the co-worker] [sic] will never complain! … But not: 'Well, for a week I have not been feeling well, and now I thought I call the fire brigade now.' Where you say: 'Well, go to the GP tomorrow or walk to the emergency department [yourself].' Or cut [in the finger[9]], or torn toenail.

Mr Leidner differentiated between cases of legitimate doubt and cases that contrasted with the 'common sense'. He expressed empathy with doubts and concerns, which are likely to match the mandate of the EMS and ED, while he expressed frustration with cases that concern long-term or mundane health problems and could be alleviated by home remedies or self-help.

Mr Leidner suggested that legitimacy entails authentic helplessness and a 'sensible weighting'. Many providers referred to strategic or intentional 'misuse' of their services, for example, 112 calls and ambulance transport requests to reduce waiting time in EDs as illegitimate, contradicting 'authentic need'; they also described a lack or loss of self-help capacities among people, which contributed to 112 calls or ED attendances for low-acute health and social needs. Mr Leidner and others delineated symbolic boundaries between patients and reproduced the doxic understanding of 'right' and 'wrong' medical paths, with focus on whether patients are 'authentic', and their behaviours are 'common sense' or not. It turned symbolic boundaries into moral ones.

The next section shows how such an understanding influenced frontline workers' demand for a narrower access to emergency care and differed from their superiors' perspective.

Working hierarchies and different positions on the width of the access

Agents in managing positions (ED managers, station managers) and frontline workers shared an understanding of their work and the field's stake, despite the working hierarchies between them (see also Maynard-Moody and Portillo, 2011, p 272). Managers and frontline workers anticipated patients may categorise 'falsely' and call 112 or approach the ED for health problems with low acuity medical needs. Managers and providers also shared an understanding of the difference between 'being' and 'experiencing' an emergency. However, depending on their position in the work hierarchy, they had different views on the 'width of access' to emergency care, that is, whether patients should be rejected or redirected from the 112-control centre or at the ED registration desk if they were of low medically acuity.

During our interview, Mr Müller from the EMS planning department said that from a 'subjective standpoint', around 30 per cent of the operations in the ambulance service do not necessitate their help and transport to an ED. Other frontline workers indicated ratios such as 50 per cent, even 70 per cent. 'But now you define what unnecessary means?!' Mr Müller asked. While he did not agree with addressing all of such 112 calls that appear low-acute, he acknowledged, 'there are people who must decide this. That means, it's a matter of definition'.

Many frontline workers saw access regulation as a form of patient education and as something for which planners and their managers had the primary responsibility.[10] EMS worker Philip explained increases are not the 'fault of people who call 112' but of the EMS not giving callers the 'chance to learn that their case is not severe enough'. Frontline workers in EDs and the ambulance service had the impression that 'every 112 call wins' and gets an ambulance, or every approach to the ED is a 'foot in the door' of hospital care, that is, to the desired help and diagnostics. The right (and need) to self-define what constitutes an emergency seems to have facilitated broad access to the field. EMS worker and crew supervisor Anton explained:

> you can see that very well in our annual reports, how the curve keeps going up … The citizen, the patient undergoes a socialization of trial and error. … a bunch of misconceptions based on the fact

> that we don't really educate people well about our work either, one thing leads to another. And so, the number 112 is dialled more and more often.

In contrast, ED managers like Dr Lindemann or employees from the EMS planning department like Mr Hansen represented a different position in the field. Instead of educating patients via regulation of the access, they proposed a wide access to emergency care services. Mr Hansen remarked:

> How is the emergency actually defined? That is quite messy. There is always this legal definition to avert life-threatening or server damage. But I think, the actual definition is quite a trivial subjective one: When my own resources come to an end! ... The subjective feeling of an immediate threat, and the lack of a possibility to self-help to put it simply. That is the subjective emergency ... and that is enough to call [112].

The wide definition of the emergency[11] that Mr Hansen (similarly Dr Lindemann) gave in our interview picks up the tension between objectifying categories and the subjective dimension engrained in the classification and techniques used to classify and sort patients (see Table 1.1). While the legal definition is assumed to produce unambiguity, the actual definition seemed 'quite messy'. And while many frontline workers acknowledged the messiness of the definition, they proposed more access regulation as a consequence (see Table 1.2).

The different work positions in the EDs and in the EMS did not determine the position towards the width of the access to emergency care, but they increased the likelihood of favouring certain position-takings on definitions and handlings of so-called non-emergencies (see Table 1.2).

The positions in the field (management/planning, frontline) corresponded with certain trainings and institutionalised cultural capital and created

Table 1.2: Field positions and position-takings towards access regulation

Field position	Training	Social exposition	Access regulation
Management	Medicine Paramedicine Public health	Peers in planning Other decision-makers	Wide
Service frontline	Medicine Nursing Paramedicine	Patients, patients' relatives Peers in EDs, EMS (and other institutions, for example police)	Narrow

Note: 'Social exposition' here refers to providers' main interaction on an everyday basis and does not exclude the potential for exchange between the levels in, for example, meetings or workshops (see Lockett et al, 2014).

specific expositions (in varying frequencies) with patients, co-workers, peers, and other fields such as public health or hospital administration (that is, social capital and professional socialisation) (see Lockett et al, 2014). In theoretical terms, this social exposition exerts influence or 'gravity' on agents' dispositions and perceptions (see Hage, 2011; Wacquant, 2016, p 67). Similar to frontline workers, managers and planners saw a share of emergencies as 'personally experienced', producing ambiguity in practice; different to frontline workers, however, they argued the EMS and EDs should be responsible for these patients, too. They argued for a wide, low-threshold access to the field. Most frontline workers favoured, however, a narrow access to their services, arguing that their mandate is clearly defined.

Conclusion

To conclude, Chapter 1 laid out three relevant aspects for the empirical analysis. First, while institutional arrangements determine paths and tasks, they also represent moral economies. The arrangement of emergency care around bounded settings reproduced doxic beliefs and moral orders of 'right' and 'wrong' ways of getting medical help. As such, the field developed a 'hidden curriculum' (Higashi et al, 2013): doxic expectation of patients knowing to 'rightly' match symptoms to medical settings, differentiating medical urgency from other complaints. The 'wrong' turns low-acute patients regularly took violated doxic expectations of the cultural category and unambiguity of the emergency.

Second, professionals reproduce beliefs in the truths and values of the field, as Bourdieu (1990, p 66) argued, through their habitus and their relation to objective structures in which a 'game' is set. The habitus is where the objectified history of a field – in this case, professional mandates, jurisdictions, standards (for example, the triage), and social positions – sediment into agents' bodies through expositions with the field (see Bourdieu, 1990, p 66). The objectified sense of a field constitutes its moral economy, which contributes to a collective belief in it and its consensual validation (see Bourdieu, 1990). Medical emergencies were of high social and professional value (see also Nurok and Henckes, 2009), and providers understood their work not simply as a job but as 'vocation' (Seim, 2020, p 66); they immersed and identified themselves with the doxic beliefs and illusio of the field.

Third, frontline workers and superiors alike acknowledged the importance of the wide access to the field to not miss an emergency; however, a wide definition of emergencies left open what an emergency entailed, except for an experienced or observed 'change in health'. Providers and decision-makers differed in their positions in how to proceed with low-acute patients as they were exposed to different sub-fields and logics.

Here and in the following, I referred to life rescue as a 'game' in the Bourdieusian sense. The use of this term may appear cynical, showing the cultural value of health and life and their professional preservation (see Fassin, 2018; Knorr Cetina, 2009; Rose, 2001). Yet the Bourdieusian concept of the field and metaphor of the game facilitates an abstraction from emergency care's cultural value to show how this field, too, relies on principles of social organisation that immerse agents, produce and distribute value, and attempt to regulate actions and relations through rules and categories. The beliefs or doxic understandings of the field are attempts to safeguard resources, not by means of overt physical, but by symbolic force (see Bourdieu, 1990, p 126). It safeguards the social accomplishments of specialist medicine which has saved many lives (see Montgomery, 1980), and thus accrued high volumes of symbolic capital. It nevertheless may be studied as 'ordinary' social field as well.

Chapter 2 addresses the 'social diagnoses' that providers and superiors gave and that concerned the social and organisational aspects contributing to the changed rhythm in emergency care.

2

Providers' social diagnoses for the patient increases in emergency care

Statistics show an increased demand in emergency care. These numbers fail, however, to capture the 'social lives' and circumstances behind them (Ballestero, 2014). Narratives and stories of providers complemented and contextualised statistics, giving insights into frontline perspectives on how and why patients with low-acute health and social problems called 112 and came to the emergency department (ED), contributing to the patient increase and constantly high patient numbers.

Social scientists often interview providers for realist accounts of organisational life, as Brown et al (2009, p 324) write. In these, interviewees provide stories on their everyday work and on the social contexts in which they practise (see Maynard-Moody and Musheno, 2003). Based on experiences and observations, providers conduct diagnoses about what is happening in their organisations, neighbourhoods, cities, or wider society. Brown et al (2011, p 939) use 'social diagnosis' for such explanations. A social diagnosis describes the 'interplay between larger social structures and individual or community illness manifestation' (Brown et al, 2011, p 939). Agents connect an illness and its diagnosis to political, economic, social, and cultural conditions, widening the lens for extra-medical factors that influence individual and community health (Brown et al, 2011, pp 939–40). I use 'social diagnoses' for emergency care providers' explanations of why increasingly more people seemed to call 112 or approach the ED to get help for medically low-acute problems. Planners, managers, and frontline workers gave various reasons for the patient numbers in interviews. Their social diagnoses are tied to dispositions and a sense for change, which exhibit position-takings, values, and what providers perceived as *normal* in families, neighbourhoods, and organisations in or with which they worked in or worked with (see Misztal, 2015, p 191).

Chapter 2 relies on *embodiment* to address where emergency care providers sensed mismatches to their normalcies in the areas they served and the organisations in and with which they worked. Those were situations in which they 'felt out of place' (Bourdieu, 2000, p 157) and in which their trust in the predictability, reliability, and legibility of the social was hurt, representing moments of *hysteresis*. Their social diagnoses of changing normalcies relate to facets of their habitus, acquired throughout life and in professional socialisation and careers. I show how the habitus is a seismograph for change. Its inertia or tendency to 'perpetuate the objective structures that produced it', stores logics and believes of years of exposition to fields (McDonough and Polzer, 2012, p 362). ' [S]ocial agents [thus] perceive the social world as stable' (Misztal, 1996, p 11), and attempt to reproduce it in its known form.[1] Frontline diagnoses were such narrative reconstruction of 'the normal'. I use the concept 'normative normalcy' (Blokland, 2017, p 104; 2019, p 108; based on Misztal 2001) for expectations of the normal, the stories of care responsibilities, and the doxic understandings conveyed in them. Frontline workers and managers saw societal and institutional changes interrelating, diminishing *normal* social support and *normal* access regulation (see Figure 2.1).

In the following three sections, I use frontline workers' and superiors' observations of changing social support within families and neighbours, organisational changes of standardisation and legalisation, affecting access regulation in the 112-control centre and at ED registration desks, and diagnoses of changing policy goals, which deviate from what agents expect as normal and legitimate. In these observations, frontline workers and

Figure 2.1: Emergency care providers' social diagnoses of increased demand

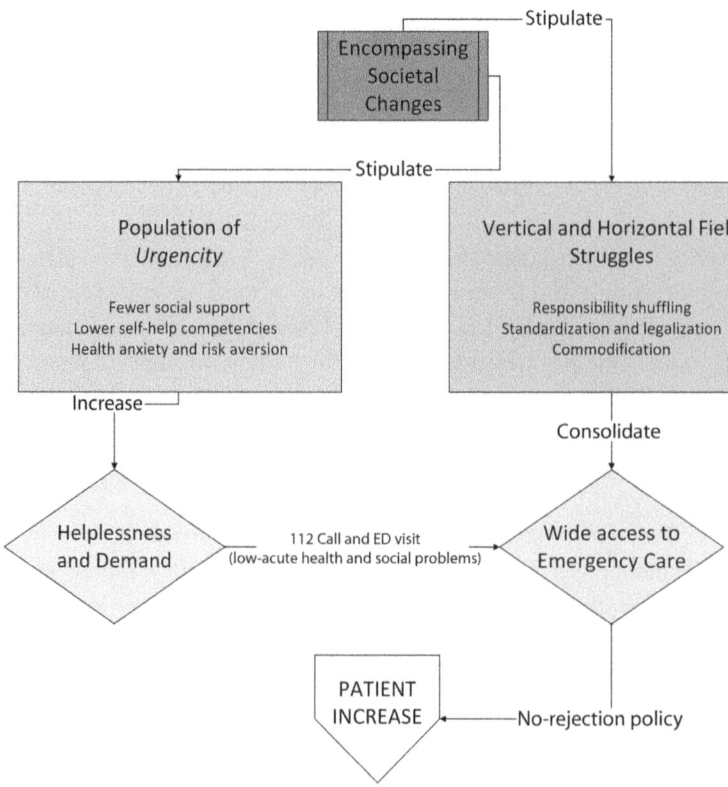

superiors convey their position-takings and engage in relational work. I use their stories as realist accounts of changes in emergency care and as relational practice that position providers and their work vis-à-vis their patients, within their organisation, and in relation to other organisations and overall society.[2] I complement social diagnoses with other research and insights from patient interviews.

Becoming responsible for older and younger patients

Frontline workers said they were 'witnessing social change live'.[3] They frequently explained how care relations within families and neighbourhoods shift and affect their work. Dr Weber described how he and his coworkers regularly took over familial care responsibilities:

> and then grandma comes with a walking aid. And this is not realistic. Of course, with a quick look, I see that grandma is not an emergency case, but how can you explain an old lady where she should go now, [or] send her away. She cannot get to the bus. She has no one who can accompany her. Hardly any old person lives in a big family where the grandchildren come along. But people are on their own. … That is social change, family structures, that's all part of it. When someone is alone at home, he [sic] calls [112].

Dr Weber suggested staff in EDs would admit older patients to the ED, knowing that 'grandma' would otherwise experience difficulties in accessing appropriate medical care outside their setting.

Research on local social support shows people rely on different forms of support to manage everyday life and moments of crisis (Wellman and Wortley, 1990). Later in life, people tend, however, to be less socially active,[4] to lose network members, and to depend on fewer social relations (Volker, 2020, p 328). Older adults depend more on their children and partners (Wellman et al, 1997; David-Barrett et al, 2016) and on institutionalised support (Dykstra, 2015, pp 5–6) than they do on friends or neighbours. Older adults often need instrumental support, such as transportation, shopping, and household chores, which requires geographical proximity (Dykstra, 2015, p 4). Organising such support then becomes difficult, as having family members in proximity is no longer 'normal' (Joseph and Hallman, 1998), and the capacity to make time for family can no longer be considered 'normal' either.

Female relatives disproportionally (made and) make time to support relatives. Chappell and Funk (2011) generally assume the need for institutionalised support increases with the increasing number of older adults, relative to other age groups in the population. The need for support is also likely to increase, as researchers suggest (Chappell and Funk, 2011; Joseph and Hallman, 1998), because of an increasing rate of employment among women who primarily provide(d) informalised care for older relatives. In short, even if people still expect children (usually, women) to care for older relatives, their employment rates and obligations complicates doing so. As an example: Mr Diestel[5] had a son who looked after him, but he could not always call him, he said, because of the son's work obligations (instead he called 112 for severe backpain). Medical assistant Eva recounted an incident where a son brought his father to the ED to look after him (with no medical indication) and went to work, picking him up afterwards. Expectations of 'who is responsible for care' continued while conditions for giving care seemed to have changed.

In a similar vein, having people living in proximity does not automatically result in neighbourly exchanges of support (Blokland et al, 2021). During a dinner break at an outskirt fire brigade station, the frontline workers described 'typical' operations, in which older patients were helpless and lacked the social support that neighbours used to provide, they reasoned:

> In such cases, nothing is said. But what you notice is that people help each other less. For example, if you go to a patient with diarrhoea because the person couldn't go grocery shopping for a while. Neighbours could do something like that, including helping if someone falls out of bed. We are catching these things now.

Station manager Mr Preiß described such operations as part of wider changes in social cohesion:

> So, in part it's certainly because the population has changed, so the civil courage is no longer there, the mutual help, maybe the social cohesion is no longer there, this family cohesion is no longer there, that people helped each other, this self-understanding has changed, this *Nehmerkultur* [culture of taking], they see us only as a service provider.

Providers, such as Mr Preiß, observed societal shifts involved and interfering with what they considered part of a past normalcy (that is, mutual help among kin and neighbours). As Blokland (2017, pp 4–5) argues, such observation of lost cohesion, community, and support expresses symbolic identity making (through nostalgia) and a perspective on large transformations that brought community and place 'out of sync', that is, largely decoupled communal practices from where people live. The 'normative normal' (Blokland, 2017) of grandchildren accompanying grandparents and mutual help among neighbours appears to have changed but not vanished. Some explained support 'still happened' (even if it generally became less), especially for socially mixed, inner-city areas, where, ED doctor Anna[6] reasoned, they could often rely on patients living in big families, providing support for relatives.

While age was a central topic in terms of care for the elderly, it also arose for younger people and parents. Dykstra (2015, p 6) writes literature on social support for older adults downplays that much support 'goes down generational lines'. Many parents would exchange money, gifts, affection, and advice with their children, until old age (Dykstra, 2015, p 6). Frontline workers emphasised the importance of exchanges that went 'down generational lines' but saw such exchanges decrease as well; they diagnosed a loss of intra-familial transmission of household knowledge on healthcare practices that resulted in more helplessness among young adults and parents for seemingly low-acute health problems.

Paramedic Lisa explained some operations could be prevented if people had more knowledge about how to take care of certain symptoms using home remedies. She educated patients with mild symptoms of, for example, a cold on alternative treatments for which they 'were thankful', as they 'were not given this knowledge at home'. Others explained how they gave patients advice on home remedies and nursing advice for their sick infants. Staff in EDs and the ambulance service took on educational roles and transmitted knowledge on home remedies, knowledge that was, as they described, 'to be passed' on by mothers and grandmothers. Anton described:

> we also notice, or [it's] such a subjective feeling ... that increased operations in the EMS [emergency medical services] are also related to the fact that people have lost a certain kind of ability to help themselves. Because they no longer have a family structure, in the past you still had a grandmother in the house, who told you, 'gee, if you have 40 degrees fever, why don't you do a calf compress, then you'll have 38 and everything is fine'. Something like that is very rare nowadays. And then I know the same extreme example in the other direction: young mothers. Are often also quite helpless and call the EMS, not because of bad intentions, but because they simply don't know any better. And in the past, such people were caught by an intact social environment, but that is no longer the case today.

Changes in familial normalcies, that is, how family members lived together or apart, exchanged support or not, and shared knowledge on healthcare along matrilineal lines influenced their work, as Anton suggested. In his explanation, young mothers appeared as carrying main responsibility for care practices, such as nursing a sick child, and their mothers and grandmothers also appeared as the keepers of domestic knowledge on healthcare, a social position and responsibility women have historically taken, as historian Leong (2013, 2018) confirms.

Dr Weber described a decrease in self-help capacities, coupled with a decrease in familial health knowledge transfer, as a current shift that influenced their work:

> And the people come – yes, these small home injuries. ... I think, yes, this decrease in knowing about corporality, so what's normal, what's not normal. What's health, what's illness ... over these three, four decades there is simply a shift to let's say less handling of things on your own ... but like, how we knew it before that you can [handle things] in your domestic, familial environment – the famous home remedies, they are still current, the calf wrap, inhaling with infection etc.

Changes in family and household composition changed the transfer of advice, as everyday exchanges of intra-familial cultural capital. Grandmothers and mothers facilitated, according to Anton and Dr Weber, the classifying and treatment of medically low-urgent symptoms that nowadays would become a responsibility of emergency care settings and their providers.

In addition to the decreasing exchange of health-related knowledge, Anton assumed online advice often replaced intra-familial advice and stipulated the aggravation of symptoms: 'Maybe you also tend to use your smartphone and the internet, to get a little more information and look for advice. ... and in all cases, it says, "call a doctor or the EMS."' Similarly, Dr Weber described that people have the tendency to 'aggravate symptoms', that is, experiencing them as more severe than they 'should' be experienced. Having wider access to more health-related knowledge does not necessarily add to people's health literacy or confidence to self-care certain symptoms at home, according to providers' observation.

Support for older and younger people for low-acute health problems, such as grocery shopping when ill, helping a person back into bed, giving advice on home remedies when having a cold, belonged to the responsibilities of neighbours and kin, an exchange of support frontline workers described as 'normatively normal' (Blokland, 2017) and as a sign of social cohesion in families and neighbourhoods that matched providers' dispositions. Through these dispositions, however, frontline workers also reproduced expectations of families, women, and neighbours – and a society worthy of their help and commitment, that is, a society in which people would help each other and only call 112 or approach the ED in exceptional moments.

Mr Leidner explained social changes increased the numbers of 112 calls and why people increasingly went to the ED, but he also said, 'It's not just society', describing organisational aspects playing a part in the changing field rhythm as well. The next section addresses how providers described and made sense of organisational aspects that they assumed to contribute to the patient increase.

High alertness and patient safety and the 'wide' access to emergency care

Not sorting patients at the 112 control centre

The EMS follows the logic of prompting immediate help. The dispatcher in the control centre depends on quickly getting information on injured or sick patients to dispatch help as quickly as possible, following so called arrival times.[7] Even when there is an ambiguous 112 call, further questioning, waiting, and sorting on the phone delays potentially much-needed help. Dispatchers are high alert which, at times, results in 'false alarms', as one of my first operations in the field with the EMS workers Dennis and Michael showed.

The dispatcher sent Dennis, Michael, and an additional crew with an emergency doctor on board to a nearby city station, where the dispatcher located a potential 'intox'[8], an unconsciously lying person on the platform, as stated in the emergency fax.[9] Following protocol, both crews, upon arrival, took out bags with medical equipment and got to the platform where, according to the 112 caller, the patient was lying on the ground. The bags included medical equipment that facilitates medical rescue, for example, resuscitation. Arriving at the platform, however, the crews only encountered the passerby, apologetically explaining he thought the patient was unconscious, but the person stood up and went away. The doctor asked if the passerby touched the patient to confirm whether he was unconscious, which the bystander denied. Dissatisfied with the passerby's response, the doctor nevertheless confirmed the 112 call as the right thing to do: 'Better one too many than one too few.'

Back at the station, EMS worker Dennis similarly reasoned, even if this had been a 'false alarm', 'you can't do anything else' but drive to a patient and assess their symptoms because, factually, 'you can't rule out an emergency over the telephone'. Despite Dennis' initial guess about the low severity of the call upon reading the fax, the logic of high alertness necessitated to encounter the patient in person to confirm or rule out a medical emergency. High alertness is part of frontline workers' disposition and habitualised everyday practice; the relevance and connectedness of this logic with the field was undisputed among them.

Despite providers' patient safety orientation, they assumed that increasing standardisation of high alertness furnished the access to their services and contributed to high patient numbers. They described a specific standardised query protocol, which dispatchers use to process calls, and which would not sufficiently select and sort-out cases. To detect and send a matching ambulance and crew, the dispatcher first attempts to collect the coordinate of the person in need. Then, the dispatcher attempts to determine the problem, and, in case of a medical problem, goes through a set of medical questions, for which callers mostly need to give yes or no responses (Sellin, 2011, p 6). With the help of the symptom-oriented questions and an algorithm, the programme determines the sequence and kind of questions and supports the dispatchers' decisions on whether, and if so, which type of ambulance and crew(s) to send.

Providers simultaneously appreciated and problematised the protocol and programme. Paramedic Ms Delbrück described taking part in a workshop for supervisors, getting insights into the dispatching programme. Although she liked the idea of the programme and what it added to the safety of patients, it had a disadvantage, as it 'completely blanks out experience', she said. Ms Delbrück continued: 'If you can't bring in your normal basic human sense, then a robot can do it, too.' Ms Delbrück and her co-workers expressed their frustrations about the programme, which seemed to restrict dispatchers' agency and to replace professional experience with algorithms.

Researchers show the use of dispatching programmes increase the likelihood of detecting medical emergencies (Baumann et al, 2009; Sellin, 2011; Mayr, 2020), especially when dispatchers stay close to the protocol (Sellin, 2011, p 6). Such programmes and protocols tend, however, to also overestimate the severity of symptoms (Sellin, 2011, pp 2–3). Thus, dispatching programmes and protocols contribute to saving lives and categorising calls as emergencies that frontline workers later evaluate as less acute on site.

Not rejecting patients at site and at the registration desk

When at site, EMS crews must transport patients regardless of how they feel about their urgency. Ms Braun remembered, for the past two or three years, the rule was if a patient 'wants to be transported, we have to transport him [sic]'. Only if patients explicitly rejected the transport to the ED, patients stayed where the crew encountered them.[10] Providers reasoned, the non-rejection policy kept the access to emergency care wide and was based on EMS planners' and hospital managers' attempt to standardise their work and be legally safe.

In the chain of rescue, providers transport patients to the ED, and if transported, ED admit them.[11] When entering the ED, with or without an ambulance, patients will be seen or assessed medically. Managers and frontline workers gave two reasons for this practice. First, patients have the 'right to be seen'. Every patient in the ED represents a mandate of action, as Dr Weber had put it. Second, as '[the] patient never comes with a diagnosis into the hospital but with a symptom', Dr Weber continued explaining, diagnostics need to be run. Similarly, nurse Tim said, 'Everyone entering the ED is seen as orange first and then triaged down', orange being the second highest category of urgency in the triage. More information on the patient needs to be gathered before a medical emergency can be excluded.

Nurse Kevin, who regularly worked as triage nurse, described not-rejecting as the 'first thing' he got told when he started working in the ED.

Similar to the EMS, nurses and doctors in the EDs stressed the role and importance of being high alert, due to the ambiguity of symptoms and patients' symptom presentations in EDs.[12] There were standard procedures like triage and other Standard Operating Procedures (SOPs) for specific symptoms (for example, for the care of a patient suffering a stroke) that ED staff knew and practised. Experience added, however, to this insight, producing what Desmond (2006, 273) describes as the 'illusio of self-determinancy', that is, the confidence to being safe that develops during professional socialisation. Work experiences and exchanges in teams teach providers that many patients who call 112 or enter the ED are low-acute and mismatch their field, so they may develop a perspective that high alertness is central to their work but not always needed to keep patients safe when their case appears low-acute.

Despite their confidence and experience, EMS and ED staff were not allowed to reject patients as part of reducing risks for patients: 'even if it goes against the grain for you and you say: "The house is full!"' nurse Kevin said, referring to the ED. Only doctors were formally allowed to discharge patients, as diagnosing and thus determining or excluding medical emergencies falls within their jurisdiction. Doctors, however, were not always likely to enforce this option. Time restraints and considerations of patient and legal safety informed the processing of seemingly low-acute cases, contributing to the wide access.[13] A patient that enters the ED with symptoms of backpain may thus be looked at differently in an ED where other standards and logics prevail than in a General Practitioner (GP) practice.[14]

Inside and outside the field, research and providers refer to the processing of seemingly low-acute patients as 'protective medicine' (see Searle et al, 2015, pp 311–12). In this reading, the intensive use of exclusionary diagnostics for symptoms as 'banal as a typical spring cold', as nurse Astrid put it, are a defensive approach to increase both patient safety and legal safety. Dr Weber explained they were 'accused of doing protective medicine', but ultimately, as he reasoned, 'a heart attack can be behind back pain'. ED doctor Anna explained they needed 'forensics' to prove what they did and how they followed standards to be legally safe. Otherwise, frontline workers may be charged with having failed to render assistance,[15] and patients are 'rather litigious these days', Ms Braun and others observed (see also Allsop and Jones, 2008; Dahmen et al, 2021, p 8). Thus, the standards that medical associations developed improved patient safety and became a means of legal protection for frontline workers and their organisations (Heimer et al, 2005). Standardisations, as Timmermans and Kolker (2004) write, also shifted the epistemological basis of medical practice from inference, experience and pathophysiology to epidemiology and risk calculation.[16]

To conclude, while patient safety is at the heart of providers' professional ethic, many observed what Mr Leidner called a 'very unhealthy categorisation' of cases as emergencies to reduce the risk of actually missing one. In their social diagnosis, many frontline workers tended to attribute legalisation to managers' position-taking (for example, 'risk avoidance') or the organisations' attempts to reduce costs and risks, while scholars describe standardisation and legalisation as part of a large shift and struggle between fields to which managers are exposed in their daily working practice (see Travaglia and Braithwaite, 2009; Waring et al, 2016).

The frontline diagnoses of standardisation and legalisation often joined with another assumed policy objective of policy and decision-makers that frontline workers opposed – that of commodification and profit in healthcare, as the following section shows.

Frontline diagnosis on the commodification of healthcare

In this section, I show how frontline workers observed how commodification seemed to affect their work. Many described 'burden shifting' or how the outsourcing of costs and responsibilities by outpatient physicians and nursing homes affected them and their work. Providers also assumed that decision-makers and managers were pursuing illegitimate political goals: 'making a profit'.

Burden shuffling by ambulatory doctors

In terms of ambulatory practices, Dr Weber assumed a 'cultural shift' in the way ambulatory doctors currently practice, compared to the three decades ago, when he was working in a practice. Today, ambulatory doctors would send patients too quickly away from their practice, without appointments, without referral to other ambulatory doctors – in other words, without giving patients orientation and showing responsibility for them, something he related to 'overload' in ambulatory practices and attempts to reduce expenses and work within their budgetary limitations.[17] Nurse Nicole explained many patients whom they triaged green in their ED are 'actually not emergencies' but cases that a GP could care for. Many GPs, she went on, 'don't do much but send patients with a referral into the ED'.

Another nurse focused her explanation on 'exhausting patients', that is, those who contact their GP several times without 'finding something' and who 'wish for further diagnostics'. Those patients also 'exhausted' GPs' budgets and are sent to the ED, sometimes without emergency referral. 'That's a stupid situation, of course, for us and for the patients. Because they think it's urgent and we don't know what they're here for because there's no referral,' the nurse explained.

Other patients are sent to the ED with emergency referral, as Dr Konrad described, showing discrepancies between what the referral states and their assessment of the acuity of symptoms. This shows the 'desperation' with ambulatory doctors, she said, whose patients would have difficulties in getting timely appointments for examinations and specialist treatments.[18] Making them appear urgent might thus appear as a way to facilitate their access to medical care and diagnostics;[19] a suggestions that research supports (Oslislo et al, 2019). Even if patients took the 'right' path in an acute but seemingly low-urgent situation and approached an on-demand ambulatory doctor during emergency consultation hours, these doctors can usually not provide examination for acute symptoms (for example, X-rays), so that an ED referral may be issued (Seeger, 2019, p 27).

Patients in search of medical care crossed jurisdictional boundaries and increasingly came to EDs: 'We have – [we] take the position that the legal service mandate is not fulfilled by the ambulatory doctors. … Because they are of course not there on Wednesdays and Fridays.' Compensating for an observed lack of provision that patients indicated,[20] EDs made use of the paragraph 116a (German Social Security Code V); it allowed hospitals to treat and get reimbursed for ambulatory patients in cases where they closed ambulatory provision gaps,[21] even if crossing jurisdictional boundaries.

Burden shuffling by nursing home providers

In a similar vein, staff in the EMS and EDs observed 'burden shuffling' by nursing homes.[22] Mr Hansen said many 112 calls from nursing homes are a result of 'deficits' in that field. Mr Weiß described nursing homes' various financial backgrounds that result in varying capacities to employ well-trained nurses. ED nurse Astrid observed that instead of employing nurses, many nursing homes employed lower paid assistant personnel who, unlike nurses, cannot conduct medical interventions.[23] She also explained fewer nursing homes cooperate with ambulatory doctors who regularly come for visits. Lower training and fewer ambulatory cooperation in turn, as Seeger (2019, p 30) concludes, increase the likelihood for calling 112 and referring older patients as ambulatory emergencies into EDs. Also, Astrid described, the patient–professional ratio in many nursing homes, especially during night shifts, is relatively low, resulting in work overload. Work overload, Astrid assumed, resulted in calling 112 and an ED transport to find situational relief, especially during understaffed night shifts.

Providers' observation of resource scarcity in the ambulatory field and in nursing homes appeared to result in a 'shuffling of burden' (Seim, 2017, 2020) or responsibility, that is, finding situational relief through the referrals of patients to the EMS and EDs (also Arntz and Poloczek, 2012). While emergency care workers also gave what they termed 'good examples' of GPs and nursing homes that cooperated well with them, aiming at issuing emergency referrals only in exceptional moments, frontline workers diagnosed provision gaps as an important factor in contributing to patient increases in their field. Shuffling responsibility means patients cross jurisdictional boundaries and suggest other frontline workers 'did not do their job' as promised. The violation of inter-organisational normalcies that other professional colleagues only refer very urgent patients has produced inter-organisational tension and contributed to hurting of the public service habitus of the helpers.

The sense of making profit on the backs of providers and patients

Closely linked to claims that resource scarcity has led to the 'shuffling of burden' (Seim, 2017, 2020) between ambulatory practices, nursing homes, and the EMS and EDs were that commodification of health care and austerity politics of the local state has increased the value of ambulatory patients. This section shows how providers assumed the city administration of *Urgencity* and hospitals to engage in 'profit-making' as another reason to keep the access to their services wide.

In the EMS, frontline workers related the increases of low-acute operations and their dispatching as the agency's attempt to gain public revenues from health insurances. Dennis and his co-workers explained that they often only transported patients who did not require treatments. These many small, dispatched operations, in which they did not spent material on medical interventions, he reasoned, 'created profit'. He and others described the transport of medically low-acute patients as 'driving taxi' or as patient transport, that is, as tasks they positioned outside – and below their actual mandate.[24]

Wolfgang argued, too, that the dispatching practice and at-site, no-rejection policy was an attempt to 'make money on their backs'. He stressed that he and his co-workers did not come to the fire brigade and EMS to 'make money but to help people in need'. This position-taking indicates the illegitimacy of 'money-making' that Wolfgang and others placed in opposition to 'helping people', a task that is not measured by profit but by whether they could provide help.

Philip explained certain agencies, such as hospitals, the fire brigade, and the EMS, naturally 'cost money', as they are part of the services of public interest – these fields could not be expected to generate revenues. Frontline workers assumed, however, deficits in finances that many city administrations in Germany faced produced a need to compensate for their costs and even 'make profit'.

Similar to their EMS peers, staff in EDs were against 'profit making'. They had, however, the tendency to normalise the need to be 'covering for costs' that their work produced. A doctor explained they never made decisions they could not 'medically stand by', but 'of course I know it's sometimes better to admit someone. Because the hospital also earned [something] and it's always safer for us legally'. Nurse Kevin wondered: 'Why are hospitals economical companies? How does a society dare to decide that? I don't understand it. Even though hospitals also must cover costs, do they really have to make profit?'

Kevin was against making 'profit based on working with ill people' but showed an understanding for the need to 'cover costs'. In a similar vein, an ED manager explained a 'relaxed bed situation is always bad for the hospital' as hospitals constantly produce holding costs that needed to be covered.[25]

Both in EDs and the EMS, providers identified 'profit-related' position-takings in hospitals and the EMS as illegitimate policy goals; the orientations mismatched their public service habitus. Position-takings of 'non-profit' did, however, not contradict the insight that costs needed to be covered, an issue that also appeared in the EMS but was much more pronounced in EDs.[26] This position related, first, to insufficient investments into hospital infrastructure by the local state, as interviewees problematised; second, it related to EDs and the deficits they produced as so-called 'cost-centres'.[27]

Conclusion

While scholars usually focus on frontline work and the evaluation of individual patients' deservingness (see Maynard-Moody and Musheno, 2003; Koch, 2020), Chapter 2 took a different angle. Earlier in the book, I showed how frontline workers evaluated patients based on for example, their individual behaviour or symptom presentation (see Maynard-Moody and Musheno, 2003, p 9). But frontline workers also evaluated shifting social relations and normalcies that influence their work: they evaluated the shifting normalcies they related to 112 callers, families, neighbours, and work in their agencies and in that of their professional peers. From the evaluation of social and regulatory contexts, providers often drew the conclusion that the fault of using emergency care 'falsely' does not lie entirely with patients as individuals. People can use explanations and blame, as Tilly (2006, 2008) described, as a relational device to draw boundaries and position themselves and others (also Zelizer, 2006). In Chapter 2, frontline workers drew moral boundaries against 112 callers for families, and neighbours who seemed to not care enough for each other.

Frontline workers also positioned themselves largely against field logics deemed external to their work which seemed to furnish the wide access to emergency care for seemingly low-acute cases (that is, legalisation, commodification). This aligns with what Schinkel and Noordegraaf (2011, p 67) describe as a struggle for professionalism, in which agents fend off influences they perceive as oppositional or external to keep symbolic power or professional acclaim.[28]

Legalisation conflicted with many frontline workers' professional self-understanding of autonomy (see also Hupe, 2012) and common-sense practice, while superiors positioned themselves closer to risk management. This again demonstrates the situatedness of professions (see Freidson, 2001; Calnan, 2015), while adding its differential understanding within an organisation. Commodification conflicted with non-profit public tasks, but, situationally, resulted in adapting position-takings by staff out of seeming necessity. Nevertheless, frontline workers, both in EDs and the EMS, used narratives about the commodification of their work which drew boundaries between them and their managements (and city senate) and pointed to the inappropriateness of suspected policy goals, reproducing occupational hierarchies and distances between managements and frontlines, forging a sense of solidarity between the frontlines of emergency care across organisational boundaries (that is, EDs and the EMS).

I used the changes frontline workers observed and diagnosed as signs of hysteresis, that is, aspects that mismatched and hurt their habitus as professional (public service) helpers. Social diagnosing reflected frontline workers' dispositions. Their social diagnoses were concerned with what changed in their city and wider society and seemed to furnish the increase in operations for the EMS and EDs for which they were accountable but for which many did not feel responsible. I differentiate between responsibility in normative terms of 'who should care' and accountability in terms of 'who cares' empirically (Hupe and Hill, 2007, p 286). Many explained operations as a shifting of responsibility and embedded their increases in larger societal changes, such as changing support in neighbourhoods and in families, and the legalisation and commodification of their work. Even if many providers explained they were (normatively) not responsible, they explained why they became anyway.

The social diagnoses rarely addressed, however, the aspect to which Holmes (2013, p 43) referred as 'structural violence', which is violence that results from configurations of social inequalities and includes aspects, such as the gender parity of informalised care burden in families. For example, several female patient–interviewees described how they lost years of income due to nursing children and sick relatives and how this resulted in poverty in old age for them 'our destiny', as Mrs Hirschauer,[29] a patient in her 80s, described the care responsibility of women. Also, expectations for reciprocity within familial or neighbourly relations can reproduce marginalisation; for example, Ms Klüver[30] explained how she had to ration her requests for neighbours for especially 'bad days' to not increase her social debts with them. Such debts for reciprocal exchanges include time, physical, and emotional efforts or money and can intensify resource scarcity (see González de la Rocha, 2020).

Frontline workers in the field were not alone in the reproduction of 'normative normalcies' (Blokland, 2017) and related diagnoses. Policy makers, decision-makers, and public discourses long have been concerned with societal changes; for example, what appears as a demise of community and social cohesion (Blokland, 2017, p 160), the technically aided categorisation of people (see Lipsky, 1980, p 198), and legalisation of social relations (see Misztal, 2005, p 190). Researchers point out that a perspective on societal change and 'normative normalcies' impairs the visibility of how community continues to be practised (see Blokland, 2017), how family relations are forged – often extending the boundaries of families of origin (see Acosta, 2021; Fink, 2021) – and how the reliance on emergency care organisations exemplifies the trust practised with such institutions (Hudgins and Rising, 2016). It impairs the acknowledgement that technically aided categorisation may reduce biases and legalisation resulted from patients' movements struggling for more participation and transparency in healthcare (Allsop and Jones, 2008; Travaglia and Braithwaite, 2009). In these 'normative normalcies' (Blokland, 2017), frontline workers shared how they saw and reproduced the social (and moral) world around them (see Misztal, 1996, p 11; Misztal, 2015, p 191). They store and reproduce this orientation through their public service habitus.

Chapter 3 in Part II will now turn to encounters: patients' navigation and negotiation of access to healthcare and providers' practices of gatekeeping which the social diagnoses discussed in here informed.

PART II

The chain of rescue: medical encounters between low-acute patients and emergency care providers

What happens when low-acute patients encounter emergency care providers at the service frontline? Part II shows accessing emergency care is neither linear and straightforward for low-acute patients, nor is providing emergency care for providers. Analytically speaking, this has two reasons.

First, while research and providers often suggest determining symptoms and knowing where to get the appropriate medical help should determine patients' healthcare trajectories, the chapter highlights the role of patients' and frontline workers' *feel for different games*. The feel for different games is part of patients' and frontline workers' experience based on their social and medical histories; that is, the socially unequal experiences people collect along their trajectories in and on healthcare as well as in and on other social fields. When patients and providers meet, they attempt to find a common ground. Finding a common ground, however, is rendered difficult by differences in their competencies and needs, and their capacities to trust in each other.

Second, when individuals fall ill or sustain injuries, they often meet more than one healthcare provider, along, what Strauss et al (1982, p 891) termed, an 'illness trajectory'. Patients thus have to work their access to services and the legitimacy of their need multiple times. To account for this and the role of varied experiences of devaluation or recognition gathered throughout patients' illness trajectory, Part II applies a trajectorial perspective (see Figure PII.1).

Empirically, encounters with the ambulatory field often precede encounters with emergency care personnel. Along the chain of rescue, the further trajectory may include contacts with the 112 dispatcher, the ambulance crew, and multiple emergency department (ED) personnel, as emergency care work is organised along a successive, temporal scheme (Nurok and Henckes, 2009, p 505) (see Figure PII.1). Patients thus need to work their credibility to request urgent help multiple times with various providers.

In the following chapters, I present encounters along the chain of rescue according to two logics: *synchronous* as single encounter and *diachronous* along a trajectory of multiple encounters. This approach allows us to, first, study

Figure PII.1: Trajectory of encounters along the chain of rescue (including prior ambulatory care)

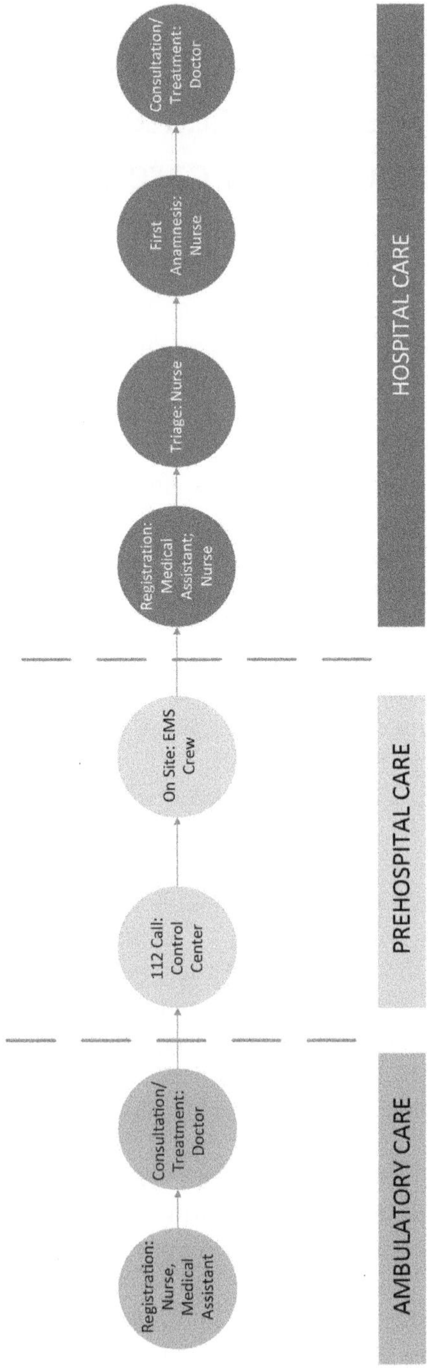

negotiations and gatekeeping at different moments in the chain of rescue as individual events between a patient of different social position and a provider of a different sub-profession (for example, emergency medical services [EMS] worker, nurse, doctor). Second, it allows us to study the work patients do along the trajectory or chain of rescue and providers' different capacities and reasons to regulate the access to their services at different moments of time. Both perspectives give insight into the processual dimension of accessing resources such as diagnostic procedures and a diagnosis – the latter being, to rephrase Blaxter (1978 in Jutel and Nettleton, 2011, p 794), 'both a category and a process'.

3

Hopes and hierarchies: patients' first step in the chain of rescue

This chapter focuses on patients' capacities to navigate and negotiate healthcare, using their reasons for calling 112 or going to the emergency department (ED) as a starting point. It uses Bourdieu's 'feel for the game' to conceptualise patients' situational trust in emergency care and their situational distrust of ambulatory care, such as their primary care doctor. Many patients I spoke to in the ED had at least one other medical encounter prior to their 112 call or ED presentation, which many patients found inadequate or untrustworthy. The chapter explores the social mechanisms behind the sense of distrust. Furthermore, it uses patients' 'baggage of history' or their different endowments, capacities, and resources (Savage et al, 2015, pp 48–9), to explain their different approaches to providers and capacities to explain their needs and express their urgency, and the associated social positions.

'Bringing baggage': (dis)trust as a form of health literacy

A common analytical model to help explaining why patients 'don't know better' when using emergency care services for low-acute complaints in health services research is the 'health literacy' approach (Dahmen et al, 2021, p 56; Schaeffer, Berens, Gille et al, 2021; Wehler et al, 2022). According to it, people are differently equipped to 'access, understand, appraise, and apply various types of health information in order to make judgments and take decisions in everyday life concerning coping with disease/health care, disease prevention and health promotion' (Schaeffer, Berens, Vogt et al, 2021, p 723). Shim (2010) argues that health literacy is part of the cultural health capital (CHC) as she theorises it; patients can draw upon and benefit from it in encounters with providers. Supporting Shim's (2010) approach, Schaeffer, Berens, Vogt et al (2021, p 723) actually show that social characteristics are associated with differentials in health literacy in Germany. In their research on health literacy ratings, they conclude, however, that social characteristics do not suffice in explaining different health literacy ratings: '[a]s the explanation of variance is low, there are presumably other important determinants of health literacy that were not taken into account' (Schaeffer, Berens, Vogt et al, 2021, p 723).

This section proposes an alternative explanation of how patients navigate and negotiate healthcare. Therefore, this section shifts the methodological focus from surveying how people (mis)match symptoms to healthcare settings, to examining their actual practices of navigating healthcare and their reflections on those practices. Therefore, it looks at tacitly and collectively gathered knowledge as 'engaged patient' (Timmermans, 2020), addressing patients' *feel for the games* as a way to bridge the 'competence gap' between patients, as laypeople, and providers, as medical experts (Luzio, 2006, p 552).

When patients interact with a provider in an emergency care setting, they bring with them a history of experiences and expectations shaped by conversations and encounters that may have occurred years earlier or only a day prior before the specific situation, and that are often based on assumptions about care outcomes and providers' intentions. This knowledge stock may inform patients' suspicions that medical professionals 'play' a different game from what they consider to be 'their best interests' (see Röttger et al, 2014, p 90). During patient interviews in EDs and during EMS operations, many patients reported having had previous medical encounters with GPs (General Practitioners) and specialists for the same health problem hours, days, and weeks previously. Their previous encounters formed part of their patient trajectory. On average, my interviewees in EDs had 1.4 healthcare encounters prior to their ED visit (see Table 3.1). Fifteen of 66 interviewees had a referral to the ED, and 51 had none, that is, they self-referred to the ED (see Table 3.1).

In this section, I use the case of Ms Schwartz, an elderly woman with potentially lower levels of CHC, and Ms Wilke, a young medical professional with higher levels of CHC.[1] Their cases are similar to the stories of others I interviewed or observed; they show how people, despite their different degrees of health and healthcare-related competences and social positions, respond with similar actions, that is, approaching emergency care for low-acuity medical complaints. Although both initially took the 'right' path by going to their primary care doctor for a low-acuity complaint, they then took a 'wrong' turn along their patient trajectories. I show how their *feel for different games* informed their ways.

'I sat there like a stupid cow': Ms Schwartz and the side effects of antibiotics

Ms Schwartz was in her 60s and called the EMS for a deterioration of her general condition, as EMS worker Max summarised her case to me when we approached the patient's apartment. After a brief introduction in Ms

Table 3.1: Overview of interviewees' healthcare encounters prior to ED visit

N = Interviews	N = Setting Encounters	Min	Max	Mean	SD
66	95	0	9	1.4	1.5

Schwartz' apartment, Max asked Ms Schwartz about her complaints and symptoms she was experiencing. Ms Schwartz explained she got antibiotics a few weeks previously, and they were giving her side effects and made her 'feel bad'. That day, she had felt dizzy and called the EMS. 'So, what shall we do now?' asked Max, implicitly questioning the medical urgency of his patient's description. Ms Schwartz responded with the request to be transported to the hospital. The dizziness she reported made it difficult for her to get to the hospital by herself. Max hesitated, explaining that the ED personnel 'would not know what to do' with Ms Schwartz, as she 'was nothing for the emergency department'. Despite Max's hesitation, Ms Schwartz continued her attempt to convince the EMS worker of the urgency of her complaints and moved on:

> I'm not a doctor, but I've seen this on TV. The tablets have strong side effects. I've already been to my GP, who gave the tablets to me, and [I] told her that I saw this on TV and that my [relative] also said that you must dissolve the side effects. The GP said she didn't know what else to do … and she wouldn't know what else to prescribe. I sat there like a stupid cow. She just let me run aground and gave me nothing.

Ms Schwartz' previous encounter with her GP disappointed and shamed her. She also mentioned having previously called EMS, where an EMS doctor had similarly assessed her case as low acute. However, convinced she was of the urgency of her complaints and the significance of the information she had received and accessed through a television programme and her relative, the providers she had encountered so far did not seem to help her access the services she believed she needed. Although Max rhetorically marks her case as low-acute, he responded to her request for transport to the hospital. During the ride in the ambulance, Ms Schwartz explained how she liked her GP and felt that she was well taken care of by her, except for 'this conflict' that had just arisen between them, a conflict in which she trusted the urgency of the information she had received and the complaints she was experiencing, but did not get the treatment she assumed she needed.

'The system is sick': Ms Wilke and her odyssey to care and diagnostics

Ms Wilke was in her twenties, had completed secondary education, and had worked as a medical provider in healthcare for a few years previous to her presentation in the ED.[2] When we talked in the waiting room of an ED, she laid out an 'odyssey', as she put it, when describing her experience to an ED triage nurse. Prior to presenting to the ED, she had consulted with two GPs and two specialists regarding respiratory difficulties over the previous weeks.

Ms Wilke described to the triage nurse, and later in more detail in our interview, that she experienced the consultation by one of the GPs as 'humiliating'. Drawing on her training as a medical provider herself, Ms Wilke said, she recognises the importance of empathy and intimacy, which she felt was lacking in her previous encounter with the first GP she approached. She changed GPs, after the first one quickly examined her in a booth that was not opaque, and allowed others to partially see her and hear what she was saying. This doctor suggested rest and gave her a sick note – recommendations she said to not trust after questioning his skill in examining her. She sought more confidence in her care.

The next GP she went to see 'at least took her time', she said, and did not 'channel her through the room like in a factory'. Ms Wilke received a referral to a specialist for further exams; however, that specialist found no need for further treatment and gave her a diagnosis that she could not trust: he concluded that the problem would 'resolve on its own'. Overnight, she experienced an exacerbation of symptoms, and she went to see another specialist within ambulatory emergency consultation hours the next day. Receiving a new diagnosis and another referral, Ms Wilke tried to make an appointment for the examination that the second specialist gave her. She called four practices and was offered appointments in three to five months in the future. 'But my problem is now,' she exclaimed, when reflecting upon her attempt for scheduling an appointment. Against the backdrop of her complaint's exacerbation, she decided to present to the ED, as she explained. When contextualising her decision to the triage nurse, Ms Wilke concluded that she had four different diagnoses from four different doctors, which appeared 'strange' to her, especially since she was a medical provider herself and was 'not drop[ped] on her head'.

Another aspect that contributed to her assessment of her situation was expressed during further conversation. Ms Wilke has worked for years in a hospital where she encountered much ambivalence between the ethics of care that she valued and the ethics that governed her actual daily work. She concluded that the 'system is sick', referring to abstract market pressures and more tangible pressures from her superiors and other co-workers to make her work more profitable and, for example, spent less time with her patients than she would want. In other words, in her work, she experienced firsthand *within the system* that providers like herself may be asked to 'play' a 'different game' as opposed to what they may have internalised as healthcare professionals and what their patients may have internalised as well. Notwithstanding this experience that might have informed her (dis)trust in former medical encounters, she expressed her 'hope to finally learn what's wrong with me' in the ED that day, indicating a persistent trust in diagnostics and competencies in hospital EDs.

Ms Schwartz acknowledged the knowledge hierarchies in the medical field, which Ms Wilke as healthcare provider challenged. Despite Ms Schwartz's acknowledged gap in CHC, she found information from a relative and a TV programme trustworthy, resources contributing to the *feel* on which she relied for healthcare orientation and that her GP did not seem to value. Ms Wilke's CHC consists of healthcare-specific training, years of work in a hospital and exchanges with colleagues. In her understanding of legitimate or 'right' medical practice, time should be taken, intimacy provided, exams conducted, and one unambiguous diagnosis found. Both patients initially took the 'right' path, approaching a GP for consultation and treatment of a low-acuity health complaint, but their differing sources of healthcare-related information and their evaluation of such information vis-à-vis the information provided by doctors conflicted with their 'feel for the game'.

Both questioned whether the healthcare providers they encountered had their best interest in mind or 'played a different game', displaying expectations regarding aspects that contribute to patient-centred care (see Timmermans, 2020).[3] As a consequence, both explicitly (Ms Schwartz) or implicitly (Ms Wilke) challenged their providers as *engaged patients* and continued the patient trajectory, hoping to receive the 'right' care in the ED.

Low-acute patients' capacities to make and be seen

People's 'baggage of [social] history', that is, their different endowments, capacities and resources, provide them with differing 'sense[s] of entitlement and authority', as Savage et al (2015, pp 48–9; 97) write. Formally higher educated people are more likely to know the right words to say to the doctor, better process and apply health and healthcare-related information and may have greater confidence in being seen for their needs and with their claims (see Shim, 2010, p 6). This section uses the example of patient Ms Gussew, who approached the ED for a rash on her foot; her case is complemented by Mr and Mrs Claßen, a couple in their 70s, who approached the ED for the 'bad impression' Mr Claßen made on his wife in the days prior to the visit. As the section will show, Ms Gussew and the Claßens navigated the eligibility to care and understood their entitlements differently.

People's 'baggage' of medical history and their resulting *feel* are related to where they are positioned in the social order. This section thus complements the former one, providing a perspective on the role of 'historically forged' social classes (Savage et al, 2015, pp 48–9) and their navigation of and negotiation in healthcare. In other words, it shows how people's senses of entitlements influence their healthcare trajectories and navigation in encounters.

Ms Gussew, who was in her seventies, migrated to Germany in the 1990s, and came to the ED with a rash on her foot that she hoped would be examined.[4] After anamnesis, her ED doctor, Anna, suggested an examination at an out-patient practice. Ms Gussew showed unease about this suggestion. She asked whether Anna would prepare a doctor's letter for her: 'If I simply go, the doctor will make me wait. If I have a letter from the hospital, the doctor will look at me differently.' The preparation of a doctor's letter for ED discharge is standard procedure for doctors in the ED. It is a protocol that includes the anamnesis, examination, allocation of medicine, diagnoses, and recommendation for further treatment. Ms Gussew's unease and explanation reflected her experience of situations in which she had not felt seen or taken seriously.

For Ms Gussew, her presentation of symptoms alone did not seem to have enough value or leverage in the field – contrary to what the benevolent logic of healthcare might suggest. Ms Gussew considered herself 'a fighter'; she was a 'strong woman' and had to 'fight her whole life', she explained to me later. From doctors who did not understand her German due to her pronunciation to doctors who gave her medical recommendations that she did not understand to the city's citizen's office and administration who did not acknowledge her educational degree, she described her struggle for accessing resources against the unresponsiveness of professionals and bureaucratic settings and how she had developed ways to respond to them. Ms Gussew integrated past experiences into her *baggage* of social and medical histories (see Savage et al, 2015) and transferred and used such schemes as a 'solution of similarly shaped problems' (Bourdieu 1977, pp 82–3 in Shim, 2010, p 3).

Different to Ms Gussew, Mrs Claßen appeared more confident but similarly 'demanding'. Mrs Claßen came to the registration desk, put the health insurance card on the desk, and explained her husband was the patient. 'Do you also want to see him?' she asked. 'Yes, that would be convenient. We still must examine him,' the triage nurse said, showing signs of confusion. She responded, 'I['ll] get him, one moment.' Mrs Claßen stepped back from the registration desk, passing the queue of people waiting, to get her husband from the waiting area, explaining to people in the queue in a confident voice, 'This will take a moment,' to ensure that no one else approached the registration desk. She came back to the registration with her husband, helped him onto a chair and described his condition to the nurse. Due to a neurological condition, Mrs Claßen, his caretaker, had to talk for him. She is an example for cases in which a relative added to the patients' capital endowment and made Mr Claßen be seen.[5]

That day, Mrs Claßen wanted Mr Claßen to be examined for dehydration. She had observed that his capacities to drink and eat had worsened. The nurse asked Mrs Claßen if someone referred them to the ED. 'Yes, me! In consultation with the GP. We talked this morning on the phone,' Mrs Claßen explained.

Mrs Claßen indicated that the decision to come to the ED was based on her own judgement and expertise, seemingly without doubting her legitimacy or authority. She explained she had consulted *with* her GP,

Table 3.2: Case comparison of Ms Gussew and Mrs and Mr Claßen

	Social position	Eligibility[6]	Sense of entitlement	Feel for the game(s)
Ms Gussew	Rather low	Uncertain	Rather low	Making seen
Mrs and Mr Claßen	Rather high*	Certain	Rather high	Being seen

Note: *Mrs Claßen mentioned aspects in the interviews that align to a higher social status by the location of their house in an affluent part of the city, their leisure activities, and their social network, which comprised professionals in leading positions.

instead of being consulted *by* her GP, which suggests an active, engaged, and collaborative relation rather than a receiving and passive relation with her GP (see Timmermans, 2020) (see Table 3.2). In her response, Mrs Claßen did not express worry that a verbally issued referral would be rejected in the ED. In this, differently than Ms Gussew, Mrs Claßen relied on her embodied capacities, whereas Ms Gussew made sure to receive, as Street (2012, p 1) described, 'bureaucratic and biomedical technologies of visibility' to be seen and thereby to 'entice governing actors to see and enter into a relationship with them'.

Ms Gussew, like other patients with low senses of entitlement and uncertain eligibility, use a rhetoric of justification and professional endorsement (for example, doctoral letter) to be seen and legitimise their claims and needs (see Table 3.2).

ED doctor Anna gave the 'fear of being overlooked' as something special with certain patients. She and her co-workers observed this fear when working in areas characterised by a high share of people classified as migrants and of low social status. In contrast to working in hospitals in well-situated urban areas, Anna explained doctors would regularly lead different discussions. There are 'fewer discussions about: "Eww, I don't want to take medication because you read so bad things about it"' but rather about the fact that they 'have to take their illnesses seriously. So, the opposite, thus: "this is important now and you have to do it"'. Another ED doctor, Dr Richter, described a 'high sense of entitlement' of patients in low-socioeconomic urban areas, indicating a perspective of patients that he related to a 'sense of falling short'. Other providers confirmed the impression that there is a general change and increase in the sense of entitlement and that patients became more demanding, observed both for worse-off and well-situated patients.

Conclusion

The chapter examined what patients lead – and bring into a medical encounter beyond an individual motive for their presentation. Research exploring reasons for the rising and persistently high demand in emergency care have largely focused on factors attributed to patients as individuals, such as health anxiety or a preference for temporal autonomy over scheduled appointments (see, for example, Kraaijvanger et al, 2016; Coster et al, 2017). The chapter began by giving an alternative. It described Ms Wilke's and Ms Schwartz's feel for the 'wrong' care, which stipulated an EMS call or ED visit in the context of prevailing, and often intensifying symptoms and worries.

Both patients initially took the 'right' path: Approaching ambulatory doctors for seemingly ambulatory-level health complaints; they then made a 'wrong turn' when calling 112 and presenting to the ED. In descriptive terms, the details of Ms Wilke's patient trajectory differed from that of Ms Schwartz; they had different capacities to evaluate and make their case when encountering providers, which is in line with Shim's (2010) conceptualisation of CHC and its social variability. In further analytical terms, however, both patients described past medical encounters and expressed what they considered as 'right' or 'wrong' when they met their GP or specialist. Employing their 'feel for the game', both evaluated the practices of providers based on their expectations and suspicions regarding medical practice and its professions which expands on their capacity to draw on CHC.

With this, the part showed a relevant but overlooked aspect in how patients navigate healthcare – employing their 'sixth sense' (for providers: Johannessen, 2018a; Wamsiedel, 2020). Neither Ms Wilke nor Ms Schwartz directly confronted their respective providers. Instead, they mobilised their information, experiences and expectations, and engaged in a process of tacitly searching for a trustworthy provider, thereby underscoring their embodied position of the 'engaged patient' – one of responsibility, rights, and critical reflection, which acknowledges the importance of their experiences (see Timmermans, 2020). In this, they exhibit their 'feel for different games' when they could not trust in the current provider, and ultimately turned to an emergency care provider with the hope of receiving the 'right' diagnosis and treatment.

The chapter's second part, accompanied Ms Gussew and Mr and Mrs Claßen and their actual negotiation for access to ED care as 'engaged patients' (Timmermans 2020) in the ED. It opens up the analysis of encounters along the chain of rescue that follows in the subsequent chapters by pointing to the differential social positions from which patients initiate and negotiate a medical encounter. It shows patients or their relatives adopting a demanding approach. While such engagement may constitute a socially shared practice, it is driven by different underlying social experiences and capacities.

From these insights on patients' differential reasons and capacities to care for their health, the next chapter will look at how providers in the EMS and EDs assess patients and their expressed urgencies at different stages along the chain of rescue.

4

A sense for urgency: providers' vetting of low-acute patients in the emergency medical services and emergency departments

Providers, too, must determine which 'game to play' when encountering patients. They draw on their *feel* to do so. Their feel is shaped by a professional sense of medical urgency, experience with both low-acute and high-acute patients, and the conditions and constraints of their work (see Seim, 2017, 2020). The following sections examine frontline workers' sense of patients' urgency during the initial (para)medical encounters along the chain of rescue, beginning with the operations of EMS crews and at ED registration. Thereby, the section follows the 'fluctuating economy', which describes providers prioritising different values at different points in time during their patient assessment (Nurok and Henckes, 2009).

Vetting for fit: the sense for urgency in the ambulance

The first part that unfolds the chain of rescue is the 112 call from which a notification to stations and the responsible or available crew results. The notification provides a first impression of the patients' complaints and condition and also includes the name, address, alarm code, as well as potential notes from the dispatcher who took the call. As others have shown, such notifications and the symptoms presented can already shape the crew's alertness toward a case and influence whether they drive faster or more slowly, or whether they carry all medical equipment to the site of operation (Nurok and Henckes, 2009, p 506; also Seim, 2020).

During fieldwork for this book, crews also attempted to derive initial impressions of case acuity from cues in the notification, sometimes relying on age, patients' home address, or details of the complaint description such as 'back pain for two weeks' or 'old fall'. Upon arrival on site, crews assessed patients' acuity with the help of the medical interview, protocols and Standard Operating Procedures (SOPs), as well as medical equipment. Providers also relied on another kind of 'equipment' they carried with them: their *feel* which stored a sense for medical urgency.

Wolfgang had been part of the Emergency Medical Service (EMS) and fire brigade more than 20 years. During a nightshift on which I accompanied him and his work partner, Sebastian, he explained his enthusiasm for paramedicine. That night, the emergency notification brought the crew and I to Mr Holdt, a patient in his late 20s, living in high-rise building in the outskirts of the city. While Mr Holdt and his wife spoke English with each other, Mrs Holdt translated to German for the crew. She called 112 for the breathing difficulties and back pain that her husband experienced.

During anamnesis, Mrs Holdt started her 'credibility work' (Wamsiedel, 2020) to justify the urgency of the call, explaining her husband had a bad cough for over a week. That day had been the worst so far, so bad that he was 'bending in pain' when coughing, she said. EMS worker Wolfgang opened his eyes widely to that description and asked whether her husband had already seen his General Practitioner (GP). Without assessing the patient, cues on the duration of symptoms and the classification of these symptoms as low-acute often informed providers' initial responses to their patients.

The formal curriculum of (para)medical training teaches frontline workers how to treat, save, and cure patients and what Higashi et al (2013) term the 'hidden curriculum' of (para)medical training. It trains providers via professional socialisation to value and expect certain symptoms, symptom expressions, and worthiness of cases along the doxic assertion of the formal curriculum. Further, the 'hidden curriculum' obscures that (para)medical practice is not based on objective criteria alone and may also rely on situational and cultural assumptions about patients (Higashi et al, 2013; also Nurok and Henckes, 2009; Wamsiedel, 2020). In emergency care, nurses, EMS workers, and doctors develop expectations of their patients in terms of pain threshold, pain response and the acuity of symptoms. In encounters, they vet their patients for fit to such temporal normalcies (expectations of acuity of symptoms) and sensorial normalcies (expectations of people's pain threshold and response). When patients like Mr Holdt mismatch these normalcies, 'another game' than emergency rescue needs to be 'played'.

Responding to Wolfgang's GP-related question, Mrs Holdt gave structural reasons for not having visited a GP. She explained their GP closed his practice, and they had not yet found a new one, describing that it was difficult in their area. In ambulatory underserved areas like that of the Holdts, such an explanation can be a 'legitimate' cause for 'illegitimately' calling 112 or approaching an ED for medically low-urgent symptoms, as Wamsiedel (2018) writes. The Holdts appeared to know the 'right' healthcare path for Mr Holdt's symptoms but experienced barriers in accessing it.

As part of the protocol, Wolfgang collected Mr Holdt's vital signs, listened to him breathing, and then confirmed his condition to be of low acuity. After that, he concluded that Mr Holdt is 'nothing for the hospital'. While the Holdts reacted with surprise to this statement (Mrs Holdt asked: 'He's not?!'), they quickly settled into the conversation and the advice Wolfgang gave: stay at home instead of waiting in the emergency department (ED) and being exposed to germs and viruses, and call the on-call service of the Contracted Physicians' Association (CPA)[1] doctor who will come to their home.

Wolfgang and his co-workers sometimes used the indication of long waiting times in EDs or the exposure to germs and viruses to test or verify the acuity of patients' symptoms. Researchers observed such practices of gatekeeping in other contexts as well (Vassy, 2001; Johannessen, 2018a, 2019b). Wolfgang later explained patients who are unwell and need help do not get 'discouraged from waiting hours and germs'. Not wanting to wait made their acuity and justifications less credible. Wolfgang's suggestion was part of his discretion.[2] It seemed to support his urgency assessment and tacitly educated the Holdts on the urgency of Mr Holdt's symptoms.

Suggesting, as Wolfgang did, to stay at home was a use of discretion in one of the first steps of the chain of rescue. When EMS workers did so, they based their justifications on 'common sense' and 'saving resources' for their service and those in the ED.[3] During my observation, however, it was more common for providers to educate patients about home remedies and outpatient alternatives, yet still proceed with transporting them to the hospital. Discretion can also be exercised in other ways: the conversations professionals have with patients, the advice they offer, the hospitals to which they transport patients, and the information they share with ED staff all contribute to the dynamics and can influence the outcomes of encounters. These variations unfold within the routines and standard practices that frontline workers implement (see, for example Maynard-Moody and Portillo, 2011, p 266).

This section used the example of a patient who consented to not being transported to the hospital and the process of obtaining that consent as an example of how frontline workers regulate access to their services by redirecting patients. EMS workers, nurses, and doctors suggested alternative trajectories that took patients out of the field. But if patients are transported to the hospital as is the case for the majority (see, for example, Günther et al, 2017), they are assessed by a triage nurse, who assigns their perceived urgency a place in the ED waiting order.

Ordering urgencies: the sense for urgency in the ED

Many patients who call 112 or approach the ED experience their situation as exceptional and urgent. When they arrive at the ED registration desk, a triage nurse assesses their medical urgency, transforming and objectifying what people experience foremost subjectively before further examinations confirm or exclude an emergency (Johannessen, 2019a). Explanations by nurses who regularly assess patients according to triage standards are used in this section to show how nurses put patients' urgencies in a context of '(il)legitimate complaints' and which role their senses for sensorial and temporal normalcies and social cues play (see also Wamsiedel, 2018).

Nurses, doctors, and EMS workers generally acknowledged the need for a low-threshold access to their services and the necessity as well as people's right to self-define an emergency. However, during triage assessment, triage nurses must also use their experienced senses to assess whether there is a (mis)match between the objective and subjective nature of patients' urgency. Dr Weber explained that an experienced nurse's assessment of medical urgency may 'come down to the same thing', comparing the nurse's habitual assessment with the triage protocol. He continued: 'someone who has been doing this for a long time has a built-in eye, so to speak'.

Nurse Catherine was an experienced nurse, working in the field for more than 20 years. She was a nurse who, as she explained, was generally cautious about devaluing patients' expressions of urgency, thereby confirming a position of high alertness. Yet the triage process included a question about patients' pain levels – an answer that Catherine, like others, regularly adjusted. With regard to applying the pain scale, which documents patients' pain intensity by asking them to rate it on a scale from 1 to 10, she explained: 'I'm also one of those, I do not strictly evaluate following the MTS [Manchester Triage System].' When asking why, she said:

> When I ask for the pain sensation, then everyone says that their backpain is at a 6 or 7 anyway. This corresponds with an orange [category]. And that would mean that the doctoral consultation must take place within 10 minutes. Instead of focusing the doctoral attention on such [low-acute] cases, they are triaged yellow or green.

To secure the 'doctoral resource' for cases with higher acuity, providers repeatedly adjusted answers to the pain scale, downgrading the urgency to a level deemed adequate. The pain scale defines certain benchmarks from when a pain relieve can be issued or a doctor should be involved.[4] In short, the number affects the triage category and, consequently, the assessment of acuity – thereby influencing the waiting time until patients see a doctor, undergo examinations, or receive further treatment. Furthermore, nurses assessed similar to their EMS peers a sudden pain, as more urgent than a long-term or chronic pain. In such cases, these patients were likely to wait longer in the ED.

Waiting created tension between nurses, doctors, and patients in the ED. Nurses and medical assistants at the ED registration desk explained that they refrained from giving patients information about waiting times to avoid being held accountable, as there was no chronological order in the ED and wait times of up to four hours were not uncommon for low-acuity symptoms (see Paling et al, 2020). Waiting times depended on the number of patients and staff in the ED and on waiting times for tests such as x-rays or laboratory results. For patients, however, ED waiting times were difficult to understand (see Fleischmann and Amler, 2014). While some hospitals began to make triage processes known to patients by putting up posters in waiting areas, the internal processes in EDs and the way the EMS worked remained illegible to most patients, and for others it did not seem to work, as they felt they should wait less for the symptoms they were experiencing. It created a limbo in which their urgency became less valuable the longer they waited.

Patients regularly came to the registration desk several times to make sure they are still in the system and have not been 'overlooked' or to inquire 'how much longer they will have to wait'. The medical assistants or nurse at the registration desk, then, educated patients on the logic of triaging which prioritises emergencies, which may enter or be transported to the ED anytime.

In a study on queues and waiting, Schwartz (1975, p 856) describes to be kept waiting, 'especially to be kept waiting an unusually long time, is to be the subject of an assertion that one's own time (and therefore, one's social worth) is less valuable than the time and worth of the one who imposes the wait' (in Auyero, 2011, p 7). Patients experienced sitting at the opposite side of the ED entrance and waiting for hours, as antithetical to the urgency of the situation that often stipulated their ED visit; some of them issued a 112 call and were transported with blue lights and siren to the hospital, which made long waiting times feel even more antithetical to them.

Nurses explained how objective criteria were central to evaluating patients and putting them in an order. The adaptation of the answers to the pain scale and the evaluation of social cues that patients exhibited influenced the ordering of cases, however, too. Similarly, Johannessen (2017, p 1180) found nurses at times overrode guidelines like the MTS, 'engaging in differential diagnostic and holistic reasoning, relying on emotion and intuition, and allowing colleagues and patients to influence their reasoning'. Depending on the patients' credibility work and whether they failed to meet the moral expectations of authentic helplessness, nurses explained they were speeding up the processing of some, while delaying the processing of others, as the following case shows.

Ms Khan – one of the cases from the Introduction – entered the ED 'by mistake', as she explained. She experienced enduring symptoms of a flu and followed an online recommendation for an English-speaking GP – a recommendation that turned out falsely, leading her into the ED. The triage nurse, Marcus, categorised Ms Khan as 'green', explaining that she would actually belong to the triage category 'blue'. This meant that Markus triaged Ms Khan higher than 'she actually should be'. Marcus clarified that Ms Khan was apologetic and well aware of the fact that she 'was nothing for this place', so he did not want to 'punish' her by letting her 'wait longer than necessary'. Similarly, Wamsiedel (2020, p 6) found authenticity conveyed in 'narrative frankness' can give credibility during medical assessments and form the basis for mutual understanding.

Nurses adjusted urgency levels of patients to account for the seemingly inconsistent information patients often provided about their urgency. For example, some patients reported high levels of pain yet moved around the waiting area, behaved, and spoke normally, showing no signs of elevated blood pressure or pulse typically associated with severe pain, as nurse Astrid[5] explained. At times, patients would use the triage 'strategically', as Dr Weber explained, to 'appear more urgent' than their symptoms were, hoping to wait less long in the ED. Attempts to 'strategically' appear more urgent violated providers' trust in patients and their need for help and hampered the workflow and allocation of scarce resources, for example, time of doctors, examinations, hospital beds, and admission to further hospital care.

Triage nurses and doctors therefore adapted the order of patients according to the medical urgency they conducted and sensed, measuring the vital signs. Like the 'vetting for fit' in the ambulance at the beginning of the chain of rescue, in the ED, non-medical aspects influenced their classification and ordering as well (see also Lara-Millán, 2014; Johannessen, 2018a; Wamsiedel, 2020). Using high- or low-triage categories and letting patients wait longer or shorter periods of time in the waiting area were tools staff in the ED could draw on to regulate the workflow and to educate patients who used emergency cues, a high number on the pain scale or came with an ambulance to gain an advantage and wait shorter over others[6] (see Lara-Millán, 2014; Johannessen, 2018a).

For patients, the processes of triaging and the order of treatment in the ED seemed to appear as a 'black box'. Because some nurses and doctors delayed the processing of individual patients, patients' doubts and complaints may be justified. Patients, in turn, may use strategic cues, demands, or even threats to emphasise or impose a sense of urgency, and to reduce waiting times, which can lead providers to view some patients' requests for help as illegitimate and indicative of an unjustified sense of entitlement (see also Wamsiedel, 2020).

Conclusion

The chapter set out the first two steps in the chain of rescue: first, encountering the EMS crew on the ground, and second, the triage nurse in the ED. Shifting the analytical perspective from patients to providers, the chapter focused on how these professionals assess and classify patients' urgency.

Emergency care providers practise in resource scarce settings, torn between a double mandate of guaranteeing a life-saving, on-demand service to the public and provide responsive care to the individual in need. They develop a sense for urgency, applied to determine how to distribute their service and which logic to prioritise at what given moment (Nurok and Henckes, 2009). For frontline workers, the legitimacy of urgency from low-acuity patients can differ by context. Patients' needs can have different 'mobilizing worth', as Dodier and Camus (1998, p 413) write. Providers practise in highly regulated (para)medical settings. They thus evaluate patients, their case, but also the options or limitations to opt for discretion, practising and prioritising certain logics at different moments – a condition of a 'fluctuating economy' (Nurok and Henckes, 2009). The first steps, such as conversations with the ambulance provider and triage nurse in the ED, set the stage for the next steps in the chain of rescue.

5

Admission or discharge: 'it's not bad enough for the hospital'

Emergency department (ED) nurses often reassess patients' conditions while they are waiting in the ED or its waiting area. This can lead to a reassessment of the urgency of their condition. For low-acuity patient, the urgency assessment usually remains stable and is followed by the final steps of the chain of rescue. These involve the assessment, diagnostics, and treatment carried out by doctors, including the decision to discharge or admit a patient to the hospital. Doctors determine whether and which examinations are conducted in response to patients' symptoms and decide whether patients are discharged or admitted to hospital departments. They formally classify patients as emergencies or non-emergencies. Diagnostics and diagnoses matter for patients as they can bring confidence and rights (Nettleton, 2006; Jutel and Nettleton, 2011). The confirmation and legitimation of 'being ill' by a doctor is a prerequisite to access treatments, social benefits, and recognition (Jutel and Nettleton, 2011; Nettleton, 2006). This section shows how patients and doctors negotiate the (in)access to such resources.

Everyday urgencies and doctoral discretion in the ED

Emergency care is typically imagined as work on bodies (Seim, 2017, 2020). Much of frontline work is devoted to assessing bodily indicators of medical acuity and addressing the underlying causes of patients' symptoms (Seim, 2017, 2020). However, another important side of emergency care concerns *talk* (Wamsiedel, 2020; also Atkinson, 1995). When patients approach the ED registration desk or are approached by a nurse, doctor, or emergency medical services (EMS) worker, these providers stimulate patient narratives with questions like *How can I help you?* or *What's wrong?* Patients, in turn, begin working their credibility: they justify, explain, and give reasons for why they need medical help in that moment. This situation puts patients in a vulnerable position: is their status of being in need acknowledged (Charmaz, 1999)?

Steedman (2000) argued that specific institutional dynamics turn people into 'enforced narrators', demanding they narrate and justify their worthiness for support or services (see also Boltanski and Thévenot, 1999). As this section will show, narration becomes necessary when patients appear to lack eligibility – that is, the specific bodily symptoms that indicate high medical acuity. Many patients feel they have the legitimate right to care in the ED, as they experience their situation as urgent. I use the case of Mrs Polat, a patient in her 30s, who approached the ED of Dr Konrad for stomach ache and with the hope of getting a specific examination that she would have to wait months for in the ambulatory sector. I show how Mrs Polat invested in the illusio of getting help that the triage nurse manifested and Dr Konrad had to violate, prioritising 'bureaucratic rules'.

I was in the ED registration when Dr Konrad approached me and suggested talking to a 'typical patient',[1] who represented the problem that her symptoms were 'not bad enough' to admit her as in-patient and to get her the examination she hoped for: Mrs Polat was 'no emergency', as Dr Konrad explained to me. After anamnesis and examining her patient, Dr Konrad did not find a medically justifiable reason to admit Mrs Polat to the hospital. During consultation in the ED, Dr Konrad explained to Mrs Polat, 'We cannot admit you. Unfortunately, this does not work.' Mrs Polat, sitting on a stretcher, got upset, turned to the side, pushed a curtain aside and started talking in Turkish to another patient's companion, who sat beside the bed and was speaking to him in Turkish.

Mrs Polat seemed desperate. She was already in the ED, and Dr Konrad had put a temporary end to her trajectory. She approached the other patient's companion, but Dr Konrad quickly interrupted Mrs Polat. She said that she was sorry, that she understood her 'problem of not getting a timely outpatient appointment' for a stomach exam, but that she could not 'admit her without a reason'. After Mrs Polat learned she was not eligible for hospital care for bodily symptoms, she raised the 'voice of the lifeworld' (Mishler, 1984 in Wamsiedel, 2020, p 5). While Mrs Polat tried again to emphasise the urgency of her situation by explaining that she had children at home and felt exhausted, Dr Konrad again expressed her understanding of her situation and the 'systemic problem' she could not help with.

Dr Konrad acknowledged a 'systemic problem' and the 'legitimacy' of an 'illegitimate' ED presentation, as Wamsiedel (2018) described the acknowledgment of contextual aspects for seeking care in EDs for medically low-acute symptoms. The acknowledgment did, however, not result in Dr Konrad admitting Mrs Polat, as she did not match the institutional requirements to become hospital admitted.

Like Mrs Polat, other patients, too, experienced urgencies that did not translate into institutionalised classifications of the suspected medical urgencies that the field legitimately served. When patients encountered frontline workers in the field, they tended to stress the 'climax' of their pain or condition (limiting the 'voice of the lifeworld', that is, those aspects without direct clinical relevance; see Wamsiedel, 2020, p 5), or described how they were 'at their limits', for example, due to high age and domestic provision issues, long-term illness, family care or work obligations, or worry for their health; some had experienced barriers to get timely ambulatory care. Many relied on justifications from their lifeworld and attempted to translate everyday life urgencies into institutionally or professionally acceptable ones. The *feel* patients show here is an expectation and trust in the professional 'goodwill'; some patients knew their symptoms mismatched those of the field but hoped a sharing of 'being at a limit' and 'running out of other options' might entice a disregard from rules and produce responsiveness with those who professionally help.

Later, Mrs Polat explained to me her disillusion – that is, the feeling of having been betrayed by something that seemed reliable or worthy of trust. Mrs Polat was disappointed with the 'promise that she would be helped' that the triage nurse at the registration gave her, as she said, and which 'the doctor did not keep'. Along the trajectory from the registration desk and first contact with the triage nurse to the exchange of her request with Dr Konrad, Mrs Polat's urgency seemed to have lost value. Furthermore, she found Dr Konrad was not a 'real doctor', as she did not help her. Mrs Polat concluded she would go back to her GP who originally advised her on the ED visit, asking him to call the hospital's department directly. Mrs Polat seemed to assume she needs to work the system differently to finally get the help she needed.

Like Dr Konrad, her co-worker and ED doctor, Anna, explained in the context of a similar case that they – as doctors – can only do 'what they are concerned with in terms of emergency care'. Mismatching cases could theoretically be admitted, but she could not 'fill the beds' with patients and their health problem that need not be taken care or examined immediately, or she would have no reserve for 'real emergencies', Anna said. In other words, Dr Konrad needed to enforce the rules at the expense of Mrs Polat's hope for a timely exam to preserve their public mandate of an ED. A central barrier to admitting patients is having a medical indication that legitimises in-patient examination and care, and on the other, 'having a bed'.[2]

The next section examines providers' use of discretion in admitting low-acuity patients, despite the institutional constraints on their agency that are intended to hold frontline workers accountable to regulations and public expenditures (see Hupe and Hill, 2007, p 289).

Practising care within and beyond the protocol

When researchers study frontline workers' discretion, they often focus on discretion exerted at the expense of patients (see Wamsiedel, 2020, p 2). When frontline workers 'stretch or break the rules' on behalf of patients at the expense of the public mandate, they 'play another game'. This section uses the case of Dr Meinhard hospital admitting Mr Müller to show that providers at times prioritise the moral worth of a case by using 'positive' discretion for patients and why they may do so.

Mr Müller, a man in his 70s, was transported to the ED by an ambulance and accompanied by his granddaughter, Ms Müller, a woman of around 30 years, who issued the 112 call. The EMS crew informed Dr Meinhard of having encountered Mr Müller in an apartment in a state of neglect. Looking at the file, closing the exchange with the crew, Dr Meinhard explained to Ms Müller she 'could not promise her anything' about his chances of being admitted to hospital due to the shortage of hospital beds. Dr Meinhard told Ms Müller they treat 'urgent medical symptoms, not chronical social neglect' in the ED.

Mr Müller's case shows how doctors vet their patients in relation to the field's temporal and sensorial normalcies, in conjuncture with the field's rules and limitations (urgent symptoms, availability of beds[3]) and also in the context of wider social conditions, as Dr Meinhard laid out in more detail in a later interview. Contextualising her admission decision, she said:

> patients are repeatedly found in their apartments in a state of neglect, who might have fell but don't have a noteworthy injury, but you still can't send them back home again. Because, yes, because you must organise it and because ambulatory – there are deficits. There are deficits, [and] there is a great isolation of older people. They have partly, really, no relatives or sometimes the relatives don't take care of it. Well, and as for the outpatient care, this can't be settled so quickly, to get a nursing care level, and to organise nursing care. And if there is no one who takes care [of the patients], you don't have another choice but to admit someone based on a social cause, so to say.

Admitting an older often alone living patient for a 'social cause', that is, due to difficulties of providing for themselves is not a rarity, as Dr Meinhard stressed later. Providers like Dr Meinhard observe the share of old and alone-living individuals growing, the intra-familial support decreasing, and deficits in ambulatory nursing. Similar to other doctors, Dr Meinhard explained older individuals became their patients due to these developments; they used their discretion to hospital admit them, assuming sending them back home would endanger the patients.

Even though patients like Mr Müller had no 'noteworthy' symptoms that would legitimise their admission, according to the logics and rules of the field, the social and institutional conditions that Dr Meinhard and other doctors are exposed to in their daily work turn the patients' 'illegitimate' ED presence into a 'legitimate' one (see Wamsiedel, 2018). The evaluation of individual deservingness and specific patient contexts and conditions can make individuals (un)worthy of positive discretion. Dr Meinhard practised responsibility, for which she emphasised the value of professional ethics, navigating and circumventing the limits of admission procedures.

Positive discretion thus was 'grey zoned'. Some interviewees explained they liked to help socially vulnerable and helpless patients. Few and certain patients benefit from the use of positive discretion, following the moral economy of the field in which specific patient groups (for example, older patients) appeared more deserving and their social surrounding did not seem to live up to their responsibilities. 'Doing good' with discretion was closely linked to the belief in these practices as exceptional to keep the field's value and not challenge its arrangement (Maynard-Moody and Musheno, 2003, pp 10–13). For providers, positive discretion did not seem to overthrow the doxic understandings of mandates and jurisdictions of emergency care, contrasting with the institutionalisation of such grey areas by policy and decision-makers in the field.

Conclusion

The chapter focused on the encounter between medically low-acute patients and providers of emergency care. It showed that healthcare utilisation and its provision are not straightforward. Many patients show engagement and assertion in accessing healthcare; they do not simply assume professionals will care for their need, yet many assume sharing the urgency they experience will grant them services and legitimacy.

Different from patients who easily prove eligible through acute symptoms, mismatching patients may feel eligible or entitled for help but mismatch the mandate of the emergency care and expectations of providers and their institutional settings. Thus, the access to emergency care is low-threshold for patients suffering medical emergencies but can be deemed of high threshold for those calling 112 or attending the ED with low-urgent symptoms. Patients may sense that. In the educating comments of frontline workers, in the hours of waiting in the ED, when observing others being treated first, their urgency appears to be devalued. Low-acute patients face the issue that their symptoms and problems are not necessarily eligible for in-patient care and are potentially of low professional value (see Nurok and Henckes, 2009; see also Palmer 1983; Seim 2020). These patients may sometimes have to put in 'extra' relational work to increase value and appear legitimate or otherwise worthy of care. Others simply give their value away (for example, in cases of social neglect). Patients could rely on differential capacities of making their claims and requests appear credible and legitimate, showing social inequalities matter in accessing healthcare, though how social inequalities come to matter is not straightforward either.

Accessing healthcare as exemplified by the chain of rescue is influenced by how it is organised. The chain of rescue shows patients may encounter several frontline workers within hours, including occasions in which patients need to work their credibility. Although it is formally the task of doctors to classify a patient as (non)emergency by diagnosis, patients already undergo evaluation in the first steps of the chain of rescue. Here, different frontline workers may 'show heart' or 'remain cold' (Seim, 2020, p 70) at the bodily and lifeworld urgencies patients present with. Frontline workers use their sense for urgencies to vet patients; a mismatch can but does not automatically result in devaluation and rejection. Frontline workers are also moral agents. Prioritising help for a helpless individual with social needs over formal eligibility criteria can follow rules of the 'professional game' and situationally be more rewarding than following organisational protocol (see Higashi et al, 2013, p 21).

Frontline workers themselves face multi-sided accountabilities (Hupe and Hill, 2007; see also Seim 2017, 2020). They navigate the poles between caring for the individual in front of them, and fulfilling a public mandate, saving resources for the team, the public, themselves in their shift. Using discretion to bend, stretch, or confirm the rules can be based on the professional worth of a case or the social worth of the patient. But a patient's case, too, can have low or high social worth. Patients may present with an illegitimate request but considering the patient's context (for example, age, homelessness, insufficient ambulatory care provision), the request can turn legitimate and be a 'moral match' (see Dodier and Camus, 1998; Buchbinder, 2017; Wamsiedel, 2020).

PART III

Grappling with classificatory change and its consequences for patients, providers, and planners

Patients often bring a wide range of expectations and needs to the doorsteps of public service organisations, as Watkins-Hayes (2009, p 31) writes. These expectations and needs often deviate from the organisation's original mandate and are thus not addressed by default. Emergency care, too, was not planned to primarily address low-acute health and social needs. While not all providers rejected or diverted patients presenting with for example, a social need when they called 112 or came to the emergency department (ED), they could not always be of help. To address the challenge of risen demand and constantly high case numbers, some organisations started to change and adapt.

The part begins by looking at the dilemmas caused by patients with mismatching needs on the service frontlines of emergency medical services (EMS) crews and EDs. It traces how these dilemmas travel to the ranks of those planning and making decisions, suggesting classificatory change. It then returns to the general underlying planning dilemma: planners multi-sided accountabilities (see for street-level bureaucrats in general, Hupe and Hill, 2007, pp 284–6). The manifestation of the 'wide access' to emergency care provided the initial access to services for low-acute patients but had unintended consequences for planners' and superiors' relations to their co-workers at the service provision frontlines and providers' relations and positions towards patients.

As the part further shows, the changed rhythm in emergency care brought providers 'out of sync' with the field and manifested a habitual lag; a characteristic of the habitus that Bourdieu called 'hysteresis' (Suderland, 2014b, p 127). The increase of cases generally changed the work demand and work conditions in EDs and the EMS; it demanded adapting dispositions to an accelerated pace, with more patients to be processed, some of which did not seem to match the mandate of the field. Simultaneously, providers observed violations of field promises, challenging the field's illusio.

The following chapters examine the social mechanisms of relatedness and embodiment, revealing how superiors and patients appeared to overturn classifications, disrupt rhythms and beliefs, and break field promises for providers.

6

From frontline discretion to institutional accountability

How do healthcare organisations at large become responsive for the mismatching needs of patients? This section starts with a frontline service dilemma. It shows how providers morally evaluated their help for some patients as 'insufficient' – a violation of their illusio of being of help. Chapter 5 showed that using discretion to help mismatching patients represented 'grey-zoned', informalised practices that produced professional value for individual cases but made this help conditional (see also Dodier and Camus, 1998). While managers often attempt to narrow such use of discretion (Lipsky, 2010, p 159; Soss et al, 2011), the next section shows how some emergency medical services (EMSs) aimed at the opposite. It also demonstrates how some emergency departments began to institutionalise care for low-acuity patients.

The following section uses two adaptation practices to show how organisational sub-fields responded locally to solve some of the frontline service dilemmas – involving patients with low-acute and social needs. The field's setup as well as the trajectories and position-takings of planners seemed to influence these developments. This part again, makes a distinction between accountability and responsibility; referring to the empirical question of who actually provides care for certain patients, and who is said to be responsible for it (Hupe and Hill, 2007, p 286).

The issue of 'circulating patients': accountability as insufficient help

This section uses the case of 'circulating patients' – those with social needs, for whom emergency care providers regularly became accountable. Providers and planners termed patients with regular 112 calls 'frequent users'. In hospital EDs, providers termed such patients 'revolving door patients'.[1] Because rescue suggests an exceptional, one-time act, emergency care seemed to be at odds with rescuing people from long-term social needs and recurring problems.

Mr Leidner and his co-workers described the dilemma of being in frequent contact with older patients in general and with some individuals, in particular. In our interview, he addressed the issue of their inadequate help that gives immediate relief but cannot solve chronic and long-term problems. Mr Leidner described their help as insufficient using the example of 'grandma

Kasulke', whom they transported for the 5th time to the ED. Grandma Kasulke, as Mr Leidner fictively laid out, was alone and unable to provide for herself any longer at home, yet transporting her to the ED where she was regularly checked and discharged from did not support her at home.

Paramedic Mrs Braun explained that co-workers from inner-city stations had regular contact with patients who were unhoused and consumed drugs and alcohol in public. She described how some unhoused patients, whom they transported to the ED, left the facility after a few hours and became their patients again:

> So, they [staff in the ED] just let them sober up for a short time and then they [patients] leave again. And then of course they carry on [consuming for example, alcohol]. So it happens that in one shift the ambulance takes a person to the hospital maybe twice in one shift, then the shift changes, they pick up the same person again, bring him [sic] back to the hospital and the hospital says 'oh, we already had him [sic] twice today!'[2]

Crews sometimes transported individual patients multiple times in one shift. A possible result of the high alertness in the EMS' dispatching practice and the chain of rescue is a circulation between street or so-called 'public scene', apartments, ambulance, and hospital for the patient group of the 'frequent user' and 'revolving door patient'. From the perspectives of EMS crews and hospital staff, the circulation and recurrent encounters produced 'regulars'. Station manager Mr Preiß described how regulars produced ambivalence: although it was 'nice to better understand the circumstances in which these patients came to live' (Krüger, 2024, p 229), regulars were also a source of frustration for him and his co-workers:

> So, I think, it accounts for most of the frustration. The colleagues are actually happy about every operation where they can say: 'Hey, here we were able to help. Here was a person that really needed to go to the hospital ...' and not according to the motto: 'As soon as we're out [of the hospital], he's [sic] leaving as well, is sitting down at a corner and takes a hit [injecting drugs] or is getting drunk or so and then we transport him [sic] two hours later.' Those are the operations we don't want and that are exhausting.

Frustration resulted from operations, where Mr Preiß and his co-workers were dispatched but seemed to be of little help. The encounters with 'regulars' reminded frontline workers of their accountabilities and limited impact to help in certain conditions. Chronical and long-term psychosocial needs of patients that often coincided with homelessness or regular substance consumption posed a challenge to the institutional logic of the EMS and EDs, settings focused on urgent conditions and acute, biomedical treatments. The same accounted for helpless patients in old age with chronic illnesses or impairments who called 112 and 'hoped for a miracle' in hospitals, as Wolfgang explained, that is, to regain health despite their chronic health conditions and high age.

In case of an addiction, providers treated patients for alcohol or drug intoxication but not for substance addictions per se or for the perhaps underlying psychosocial conditions, turning patients, as Anton[3] described, into 'a cue ball in the system' (Krüger, 2024, p 230; Krüger and Schuster, 2025, p I/26). Some patients encounter regular institutional help which seems to 'bandage' deeper social injuries and wounds without healing them (Krüger, 2024, p 230; also Watkins-Hayes, 2019; Seim, 2020), indicating the field's situational limits. Shortage in capacities at hospital departments impaired on the options to issue responsive, long-term support for circulating patients. Eventually, as Anton suggested, the collective achievement of the field's immediate help and low-threshold access resulted in logics that turned institutionalised care into a 'vicious circle' of repeated encounters – transports to the ED and discharge onto the street – from which providers and patients seemed to 'not get out'.

Mr Reimann of the EMS planning department added that other government agencies and the public could 'look the other way', which means, ignore the circumstances of certain patient groups, such as unhoused individuals and of those consuming on the streets who prolong infections, while they could not; they were being held accountable for problems they could not immediately solve. Mr Reimann suggested that even EMS was not 'really looking' at the systemic problems they were encountering with certain patient populations. They were transporting people, sometimes several times in one shift, for whom the ED might not be able to provide adequate institutional and social support.

As Biehl (2012, p 251) argues, the paradox of institutionalised care may be that it suggests 'care' but is at times experienced as the opposite: social neglect and collective 'disregard' (in Krüger, 2024, p 222). Providers in the EMS and hospital staff questioned the benefit their regulars or particular patient groups had from the recurring encounters with them. Anton said 'their hands were tied' in terms of making a difference: narrow protocols and mandates gave little room to manoeuvre, except for singular practices of discretion. Many circulating patients mismatched the field and had frequent contact with frontline workers, which broke with the field's illusio of rescuing and being of help.

The descriptions of providers showed ambivalence: they often felt they were of little help when confronted with circulating patients and their social needs. At the same time, narrow protocols and mandates were a resource, in terms of drawing boundaries between responsibilities.

Institutional responsiveness with mismatching patients

Since 2015, Germany has been engaged in an intensive debate about reforming emergency care. In 2024, a draft bill for such a reform was presented but ultimately failed to reach a vote in the then government (Bundesministerium für Gesundheit, 2023; 2024a; 2024b). Following the dissolution of the previous government, the new government initiated new negotiations in 2025. In this, one of the key elements is the establishment of an alternative ambulatory care structure alongside EDs, designed to treat patients with low-acute health needs (Bundesministerium für Gesundheit, 2025). Without the reform having passed, some EDs already opened such practices during the research period (Baier et al, 2019).

Contracted Physicians' Association (CPA) outpatient doctors staffed these practices during hours and days when regular outpatient care was closed. Patients identified by intake staff as suitable for ambulatory treatment were redirected to the on-call ambulatory doctor. While some of my respondents expressed caution about the potential beneficial impact of this arrangement on relieving ED patient numbers, others were critical and saw it as a way of offering patients greater convenience. Most of the doctors and nurses I spoke with, however, welcomed the approach. It promised greater responsiveness to patients and lower burden on ED staff.

Implementing a new arrangement of the EMS by law was more complicated (Berger et al, 2024). The federal states' EMS were not part of the German Social Code V, which regulates the health care system and its planning. Policy makers still debated whether to integrate the EMS as part of the healthcare system.[4] In response, EMS throughout Germany developed local arrangements. The EMS in Berlin, Oldenburg and further German regions, for example, developed classifications beyond the biomedical model of health and illness to account for the case increase and to better accommodate patients with low-acute health and social needs (see Krüger and Schuster, 2025). In 2019, the 112 EMS hotline in Berlin also developed an interface with the hotline of the on-call CPA ambulatory doctors (116 117) to refer low-acute patients to the ambulatory care sector (Breuer et al, 2024). How does change of this kind come about within an organisation? While institutional leeway is one important aspect, another seems to be agents with experience of working at the service frontline who also work in planning.

Mr Hansen was part of the EMS planning in *Urgencity* and also considered the potential benefits of widening the institutional responses of emergency care. He used to work as a frontline service provider in the EMS before working in planning. When talking about inadequate help for 'circulating patients', Mr Hansen recalled a 'turning point' in his work. During an operation, he talked to a neighbour of a patient with low blood sugar level whom the daily nursing service regularly found unconscious at home; a neighbour told Mr Hansen the EMS had been to the patient multiple times in two weeks. Mr Hansen thought, '"Gee, you've got to tell that to the GP." … in the interest of the patient, but also in the interest of the economy!' Mr Hansen attempted to call the patient's GP to suggest a more intense nursing level for the helpless patients. Attempting to reach out to the GP, he found himself confronted with the 'very fragmented healthcare system'. Mr Hansen unsuccessfully attempted to help the patient by organising the care they appeared to need. He described how such incidents confronted him with the limits of his professional capacities that later informed his work in planning.

Dilemmas in service provision are not documented in protocols or statistics; only frontline experiences captures them (see Lara-Millán, 2017, p 93). While researchers widely applied the scholarly explanations of institutional diffusion (a scholarly position of the neo-institutionalism; see Wang, 2016), this section relates to the agents' professional trajectory, position-takings, and field struggles to contextualise organisational changes. Some of the employees were trained in public health[5] and thus exposed to doxas of other fields, extending the biomedical model of health and illness (for example, position-takings of public health struggling over the dominance of biomedicine, see Collyer et al, 2015, p 690).

For Mr Hansen and the planning department, the 'biopsychosocial model'[6] of health and illness appeared 'very very valuable' for emergency care, he said. He explained how EMS in Germany and, for example, in Denmark, piloted services that respond to patients' social and low-acute health and nursing needs; for instance, ambulances offering nursing care such as the Community Paramedic (Seeger et al, 2021; MDR, 2023), social care units like the Sociolance in Copenhagen (Kristensen et al, 2018), or social case management services in Berlin (Breuer et al, 2020). Similarly, studies explore the need for social work in EDs (Gordon, 2001; Ruegenberg et al, 2024; Rieder, 2025).

While the use of discretion described in this book demonstrated responsiveness to individual patients and their needs, providers also often invoked professional boundaries, emphasising the responsibilities of families and neighbours, as well as the institutional mandates of social workers, nursing facilities, and crisis intervention teams. The differing position-takings between providers and planners reflected underlying concerns about what their respective professions 'should' encompass. Many providers advocated for a 'repurification' of their profession, while Mr Reimann from the EMS planning concluded they have not 'moved away from [their profession], but much has been added to [it]'. He continued:

> And here we are again at the point, what profession do we stand for? And yes, our profession is still, it happens again and again that we

> rescue people out of burning houses. That we get people from under a subway train. And that we reanimate people. But that's not all it is. And that's not the big picture anymore!

Mr Reimann later enumerated stakes added to their field, describing a ratio from fewer operations that include fires and life rescue and a large share of operations that include social support, nursing, and ambulatory healthcare needs, raising the question of how their organisation is supposed to respond to these calls and operations.

Conclusion

The chapter demonstrated how the field of emergency care in Germany and internationally started to develop institutional responses that pilot care for low-acute patients and those with psychosocial needs. This represents a paradigm shift. Piloting new structures involved in part institutionalising pragmatic solutions previously found 'on the streets', as well as discretionary practices of providers. In some cases, it entailed the integration and coordination of health and social services.

The case of a former frontline provider who later worked in planning showed how the dilemma of providing 'insufficient' help to some patients extended into the realm of planning and decision-making, illustrating how exposure to frontline dilemmas and agents' position-takings may shape institutional responses.

If these pilot services were to become regular organisational programmes, this would manifest a 'widened access' to emergency care with the formal addition of new 'stakes' in the field. At the time of the research, however, new structures remained limited to pilot studies. Many providers already understood the prevailing set-up of the field as unregulated, 'wide' access. The next chapter will show how providers responded.

7

Accountable to patients or coworkers at the service provision frontline? The zero-sum dilemma of planners

This chapter considers how patient cases and working conditions serve as potential sources of symbolic recognition and social support for providers at the service frontline. The analysis reveals that maintaining low-threshold access to emergency care had a downside: it made it more difficult for providers to feel valued by their superiors and to maintain confidence in the skills and experience they had developed over years of practice.

Exhaustion and shortage: the experienced 'lack of care' for the service frontline

With the increase of patient numbers in emergency departments (EDs) and the emergency medical services (EMS), providers in *Urgencity* experienced a higher job demand, with physical and emotional strains and less investment and time to help low-acuity patients and socialise with colleagues. Many frontline workers attributed at least part of the changes and their circumstances to superiors and planners, whose position on the width of the access to emergency care many disagreed with (see Chapter 1). Some providers from EMS and the fire brigade have brought these conflicts to public attention or addressed them internally. While scholars often interpret such responses as struggles over working conditions, this section suggests understanding them as expressions of a perceived 'decline in care' for providers at the service frontline.

Between 2017 and 2023, emergency care personnel and their representatives debated and protested developments in their field in Germany and beyond (see, for example, Hölter, 2018; Bündnis Pro Rettungsdienst, 2022; Rettet den Rettungsdienst, 2022; Deutsches Ärzteblatt, 2023a, 2023b, 2023c). There were protests in *Urgencity* as well.[1] Paramedic Ms Braun explained her co-workers initiated protests in *Urgencity* to draw attention 'to problems and circumstances in the agency and their working environment'. Among other things, they pointed to poor general conditions of stations and equipment and a lack of public investments into their infrastructure and into what providers considered their central stake: public safety. Frontline workers directed the protest and demands against their superiors and the public institutions that provide funding. Central to the protest, as Ms Braun described, the EMS in *Urgencity* had 'too little personnel' for 'exorbitantly high numbers' of operations. EMS worker Philip explained many frontline workers who already worked 20 to 30 years in the EMS and fire brigade were frustrated, as they witnessed 'the great saving' in equipment and recruitment of staff. The funding, staffing and equipment did not proportionally adapt with the rising patient numbers, he and others explained.

While during the research period for this study, hospital staff did not yet publicly protest,[2] doctors and nurses expressed their sympathy and support for the protest in the EMS and fire brigade. In hospitals, doctors and nurses described how austerity politics added to the strain in the field, including hospitals. Mr Kemper explained that public investments in hospital infrastructures often did not cover hospital investment costs. Nurse Catherine described, 'We used to have a better ratio of nurses and fewer patients. So, that's actually absurd. … Today, we have fewer personnel and the double of patients compared to 10 years ago.' She described her shifts often feeling 'like a marathon', with few moments left for her to breathe. The development of numbers of staff in EDs, as Riessen et al (2015) pointed out, did not grow proportionally with the increases of patients in the respective settings. Scholars similarly suggest cost-containment efforts in German hospitals have led to inadequate staffing and high workloads (see Dück, 2022, p 17; Wendt and Thompson, 2004).

Personnel shortage and high workloads had implications for other parts of the work: it led to higher fluctuations in ED teams and relocations of personnel with specific paramedical trainings to meet operational concepts. The management 'broke' some colleagues, Philip said, using the example of an 'uprooted colleague', who was taken out of his social environment and relocated from his station, after working there for 20 years. In hospitals, staff fluctuated as well. A nurse who recently changed to another hospital said all hospitals 'attract with great offers'; she changed her workplace hoping conditions would be better between hospitals but soon gave up that hope: 'But really, it doesn't matter where you are. The conditions suck everywhere,' she concluded.

Fluctuation influenced the cohesiveness of teams and trust in each other's competencies, as several nurses explained. Generally, frontline workers established supportive relationships and confidence in teams and developed obligations towards each other over years; relocation and fluctuation can disrupt moral economies of support and dept, as Henckes and Nurok (2015, p 1033) explain.

Many experienced the changing job demand and relocations, as in case of the fire brigade, as a 'lack of care' from superiors. While nurses can be autonomous in choosing hospitals close to their homes, frontline workers in the EMS and fire brigade are relocated according to operational concepts and demands.[3] For some, this meant longer commutes and reduced the amount of time at their disposal and with that a crucial resource, as Strazdins et al (2011, p 545) argue, for investments and exchanges in other social fields (for example, friendships, family, and teams). Additionally, the increase in patient numbers and disproportional staffing led to working overtime.[4]

Mr Weiß said the management has a 'duty of care' towards their employees to rest while on call, a duty with which superiors would not always comply. In EDs, staff did extra shifts and overtime, which let to exhaustion, too. Kevin described how certain shift schemes should apply to them, giving enough time for rests between blocks of shifts, but due to personnel shortage and colleagues choosing shifts 'more egoistic', such schemes would often not work out, giving less time for rest and a private life, as one of his colleagues added. 'Sure,' he said, 'we have chosen the profession for ethical, social reasons. I want to help people, but at what price? Not under these conditions!' Instead of supervising the adherence to working hours, Kevin said hospital managements 'liked it' when nurses and resident doctors: 'sacrifice and are idealistic, stay longer [hours], or live here in a way. … but there must be another way! The system must not be based on this!'

Intensified work demand resulted, as some described, in more sick leaves and illnesses among many frontline workers, especially those with ample work experience. During field stay, I accompanied and talked to frontline workers with 20 to 30 years of work experience, and they described mental and physical health problems (see Hering and Beerlage, 2004). High patient numbers can add to already existing exhaustion (see Karutz et al, 2013). The exhaustion that providers described seemed to lead into a 'gigantic level of sick leaves' among co-workers in the EMS and fire brigade, Mr Weiß said. In EDs, too, ED managers and head nurses who organise work schedules described absenteeism and sick leaves they attributed to exhaustion and job demand. Increases in cases made working in EDs more 'unattractive', as head nurse Astrid explained. Generally, the workload influenced how much time providers could rest and invest into other social fields such as friendships, family or sports, and how appreciated they felt by superiors.

Frontline workers' sense of distrust in their competencies

This section uses the case of the implementation of a new training as paramedic and the different spaces to manoeuvre and reject patients in EDs and the EMS to show how non-doctoral providers related their options to 'reject patients' with recognition and trust in their competencies.

While nurses were not allowed to reject patients in the ED, some ED managers stressed the competencies experienced nurses had in evaluating patients' medical urgency, giving them discretion in advising 'trivial' – seemingly low-acute – patients to take another medical path (see also Vassy,

2001; Johannessen, 2018a, 2019b). Managers described recognising nurses' competencies by practising 'flat hierarchies' and involving nurses in decisions over medical treatments and, situationally, giving them competencies that 'reached into the doctoral profession', as nurse Nicole described. Flat hierarchies and showing trust in nurses' competencies were key for valuation and keeping personnel, Dr Lindemann and Dr Weber explained; however, trust given to nurses in advising patients to take another medical path differed among the ED managers.

In the EMS, the space to manoeuvre was narrower. Frontline workers used to decide rejections and transports, as Philip explained. But this changed years ago. 'These days', as Philip said, in the EMS, only doctors can 'formally reject'. The right to diagnose rested with doctors whose medical training was aligned and certified doctors for such tasks. Superiors and decision-makers placed their institutional trust in doctors, making them the only occupational group in the field who, by jurisdiction, could distinguish between medical (non)emergencies.

The not-rejection policy appeared to limit professional autonomy for EMS workers. 'You're just a stupid handyman. Let a doctor decide,' Philip mimicked the assumed standpoint of superiors and described what he and others experienced as devaluation of their competencies. Standard Operating Procedures (SOPs) and their effects reduced abilities to manoeuvre, Philip explained, had 'much to do with trust. … Because, in the end, it is – what I notice that [those] from above don't trust in our work anymore.' Later in the interview he added:

> I don't think that the people above [superiors] are aware of why so many people are opting out. Because they really think they [providers] don't want to do it anymore. And that's really not true. Okay, the one or the other is among them who is really upset, but that's also a sign of frustration. Where does it come from? How do you actually treat people! And I simply tell myself: trust! Trust in what I teach them!

Philip linked trust to care. According to him, the frustration and disappointment experienced by him and his colleagues stemmed from a lack of confidence in their superiors. The growing regulation of their work, especially in dealing with low-acute cases, was perceived as a sign of distrust in their ability to classify patients – skills that, he described, had been taught to him by the agency and manifested over many years of practice. As restrictions on re-directing or rejecting patient transports manifested, the experience and training of EMS workers – their cultural capital – lost value in comparison to that of the higher-ranked professional group: medical doctors.

In addition to the experience of diminishing autonomy, experienced providers in the EMS and fire brigade described undergoing new training and facing the consequences of having their competencies devalued. In 2013, Germany introduced the federal Paramedic Act[5] and with that a paramedic training that replaced lower-ranked, EMS worker training. According to this act, all frontline workers of a specific status group had to undergo paramedic training. The legislator set a duration of ten years (2016–26), during which lower-ranked EMS workers were allowed to practise emergency care without training as a paramedic.

A generational divide showed in the evaluation of this changed arrangement. Younger, already trained paramedics, such as Ms Braun, welcomed the training and its qualifications, describing the advancements in patient safety, their gains in paramedical competencies, and their own position as assisting doctors on site. Younger paramedics experienced the higher-status paramedic training as valuation of their position. In contrast, many experienced providers considered an advanced paramedical training as not necessary. Station manager Mr Timmermann said his experienced co-workers were already well trained when becoming a lower-ranked EMS worker, making further training appear unnecessary. He said: 'We used to rescue people and we rescue people today. No paramedic [training] would have been necessary for this. We can do it now as we did then, still the colleagues need to go through this [training].' Mr Timmermann was concerned about the additional workload the training produced for his co-workers.

In a group discussion among EMS workers, including firefighters and paramedics, providers voiced their hope that the planning department would 'have their backs legally' and 'stand behind their personnel', thereby enabling them to reject what appeared to them as unnecessary transports. Beyond the inability to reject cases, providers experienced a differential (de)valuation of their competencies, which contributed to their disillusio. Many viewed the non-rejection policy and the new training as a broken promise; a shift in which superiors appeared to replace trust in their expertise with a focus on legal safety (a more general shift described in Misztal, 2005). It contributed to a discrepancy between competency and practice, as the following section expands on.

The frontline discrepancy between theory and practice

Emergencies are emotionally and physically the most challenging cases (Hering and Beerlage, 2004); but in terms of professional value, they can also be the most rewarding (Henckes and Nurok, 2015, p 1033). Providers engaged in exhausting training and regularly experienced challenging operations. Superiors and trainers prepared them with training, equipment, and mandate to rescue, and rescued patients were 'incredibly thankful', as ED doctor Anna put it. To the challenge and demand of life rescue, the high numbers of patient and particularly the low-acuity cases, however, produced a discrepancy between field illusio and everyday work. Frontline workers explained this to be a hurtful situation.

While the demands in competencies were high in the EMS and EDs, many patients whom providers cared for seemed to contradict the trainings and professional value. 'Never in my life have I been so well trained and was so rarely needed in operational service because what I do is actually *Pille Palle* [colloquial for trivial situations],' EMS worker Philip concluded. Wolfgang, who repeatedly expressed his genuine interest in EMS work, described, 'The many unnecessary operations are demotivating' and 'hurtful'. He said, 'This has nothing to do with prestige and recognition,' relating to both superiors and 112 callers. Nurse Evelyn said she did not train to become an emergency nurse to nurse but to rescue: 'A master craftsman would not come to change a faucet either,' she said while reading a file of a patient who was admitted for a seemingly low-acute health problem.

Low-acute patients, as supervisor Mr Leidner described, contributed to providers' disengagement with the field:

> I'll tell you right away that the biggest problem [in terms of] what is a burden to the co-workers! We're not talking about the physical strain but the psychological strain. On the one side the training, the quality [of training] is ramped up, but what ... drove them to start here: 'I want to save lives, I want to help. I want to help where others can't, and I want to be first responder and devote myself!' This is taken from them because they transport garbage! And this discrepancy in the head, this makes sick! It brings you down!

Engaging with low-acute patients seemed to contradict training and competencies of providers and produced a hurtful theory–practice discrepancy. Philip concluded the current arrangements in the EMS system, based on increasing 'understanding for patients' and decreasing 'understanding for them'; 'that's what's upsetting many of the people [co-workers] here'. Discrepancies can produce a feeling of hysteresis. People express a lag between habitus and field in frustration (Margies, 2021, 2024). The lag can manifest in illness and disengagement (McDonough and Polzer, 2012), as Mr Leidner suggests and the next chapter expands on.

Conclusion

Consolidating a wide access to EMS and ED services had a downside: in both settings, providers observed growing resource scarcity and rising job demands. This chapter demonstrated the symbolic dimension of these developments. Increasing workloads and inadequate resourcing, combined with diminishing autonomy, were experienced as a form of devaluation by superiors and planners, undermining what providers habitually stood for as 'helpers'. Autonomy plays a key role in sustaining the symbolic value of professionals, reinforcing trust in both their formal competencies and the experience gained over years of service (Hupe and Hill, 2007, p 282). Instead, providers perceived a decline of recognition for themselves and their needs, while more attention seemed to be given to patients. Superiors and patients appeared, in their eyes, to align in breaking the field's implicit promises: to be cared for, trusted, acknowledged as professionals, and equipped with the means to rescue.

8

The changing 'game' of emergency care: hysteresis and disillusio at the service provision frontlines

Organisational changes can disrupt how workers make sense of their roles and the reasons behind their work (Lockett et al, 2014). With that, established ways of being and knowing are called into question. A mismatch between habitus and field – hysteresis – can emerge, leading agents to disengage from the field through disillusio. This chapter illustrates how providers perceived violations of their professional standards and devaluations of their position by patients, deepening their disillusio. These experiences undermined their dispositions as helpers, appeared to affect their health and well-being, and led some to disengage from and ultimately leave the field.

Moral injuries: 'not helping patients, not serving society'

A strong caring ethic makes providers prone to what scholars have termed 'moral injuries', that is the conflicting feeling of producing 'unnecessary patient suffering' due to working circumstances (Čartolovni et al, 2021, p 594). A moral injury occurs when providers cannot practise their work according to their standards or ideals, observing or assuming suffering of others (see Čartolovni et al, 2021, p 595). Analytically, moral injury resembles a violation of the field illusio and disposition as helper. It can result in disengagement. McDonough and Polzer (2012, p 366) show how organisational restructurings in public service emotionally disengaged frontline workers from jobs and from 'their taken-for-granted ways of being a "good" public servant' (McDonough and Polzer, 2012, p 357) who serves the common good.

In the field of emergency care, nurses and doctors explained how illness, sick leaves, fluctuation in teams, and certain demeanours with patients and colleagues showed their disengagement. Nurse Kevin experienced moral injuries due to conditions in which he was supposed to provide care for patients. He answered my question about nursing patients according to his professional ideals:

> No. So, I don't have the opportunity to implement in everyday life what would actually be my wish. I motivate myself simply by saying: 'I try to do

> the best possible with the resources I got' and I have a compartmentalisation mechanism, [so] that I say: 'Of course it is not necessarily human and nice but I'm not the person who awards this woman with 5 minutes! I can try to make the best out of these 5 minutes …'

Working conditions as, Kevin described, limited his capacities to give patients the care he was trained to give and would like patients to receive. This limitation had also to do with how emergency departments (EDs) are planned: because the ED is a station through which emergencies are supposed to quickly pass before they are distributed to matching hospital departments, crowding, and difficulties in finding bed space increases the time patients spend in EDs. Nurses reported not having the space and means to nurse patients adequately in the ED. Kevin like others could rarely feed, wash, nor make patients comfortable. He said he learned after he finished training, he had to 'perform theatre', not having the capacities to uphold the standards he learned in his actual work. Other nurses and doctors described how the sight of suffering and uncomfortable patients in the ED made them 'feel sorry', but they did not have the space, means, time, or emotional capacities to serve patients during peaks, according to what they considered their caring standards.

Providers in the emergency medical services (EMS) also experienced moral injuries. EMS worker Philip who worked in the EMS and fire brigade for around three decades said they could 'not meet their standards anymore'. The increasing 112 calls and dispatched operations burdened the system. A 'system that used to work doesn't work anymore', he said, problematising the dispatching practice and operational management. The assumption to not be able to meet arrival times for acute cases due to the system's strain produced moral injuries. Philip said because they do not reject calls, resources are bound which may lead to 'patients waiting longer for an emergency doctor which may harm them'. Mr Leidner described the 'double story' of being bound to a low-acute case, whereas the emergency 'around the corner waits to be served by an ambulance from further away'. It frustrated and wore out co-workers, as Anton and Ms Braun explained.

An EMS worker described 'doing the splits' to keep the EMS service and first aid functioning despite rising patient numbers and what he saw as inadequate staffing. A nurse spoke of a 'balancing act on ice', juggling multiple responsibilities under time pressure such as triage, administering intravenous (IV) treatment, registering patients, answering phones, and preparing in-patient admissions. Both nurses and doctors pointed to the risks associated with high workloads, crowded EDs, and packed waiting rooms. This situation violated their illusio, that is, the deeply held belief in their role as helpers – while the continuous and often overwhelming patient demand for help further contributed to their disillusio.

Demanding help: helpers as 'service providers'

In addition to the rise in patient numbers, providers also observed a shift in patient behaviour: rather than asking for help, patients increasingly *demanded* it. Partly enforced by threats, insults or physical aggression, the emerging position of patients as 'entitled' to help marked a shift to being a 'service provider', as paramedic Leyla suggested. It contributed to the effect of disengagement from the field. Mr Leidner explained insults and physical aggression from patients 'reinforced the effect' of frustration. His co-workers would ask themselves, ' [W]hat did I actually do this for?' He found the 'appreciation for them got lost', an observation that many others in the field shared.

ED doctor Mr Kemper said, '[p]atients have a supposed entitlement. "I want to have everything checked up in a possibly short time!" This is, of course, something they find in the field of emergency medicine.' His co-worker, Dr Richter, added the service attitude is part of a 'current Zeitgeist'. Providers saw patients' desires for time autonomy to match the 24/7 availability of emergency care and a sense to entitlement to that care. Patients sometimes enforced their entitlement with threats, as Max explained. He recounted a recent shift in an ED in which he successively cared for several acute patients:

> I couldn't get out of the shock room.[1] We had several polytrauma in a row. Then, I walked out the door once and a patient approaches me [asking], why he's still waiting. I say that we had several emergencies and that I can't take care of his needs [right now]. And then he said: 'That's outrageous! He came after me!' So, you can't think of anything to say. ... It's the same for the EMS. ... [Recounts a low-acute case] And then [when] you say something that they also could have taken a cab, people quite cheekily say: 'You must drive me! I insist!' That gets you down, and you must drive them. They take down your name and the number of the ambulance and say they're complaining.

Demanding patients without understanding of the work that providers do, its logics, and stakes and threats by patients were a disappointment for many. Providers said they 'had to' transport and provide care, violating the moral economy of the field. Scholars argue, moral economies that regulate the exchange of help based on patients asking for help, presenting themselves as deserving and helpless, and being thankful (Fassin, 2008; Huschke, 2014; Ticktin, 2017). It is part of the historically grown relationship between professionals and service clients (see Steedman, 2000). Supposedly 'entitled', 'threatening', and 'aggressive' patients violated these expectations and, in doing so, disrupted the illusio of the field and its professions. These patients appeared to break the implicit promise to appreciate and respect those in helping professions for their commitment and sacrifices (see Fassin, 2008).

Providers in the EDs and the EMS concluded they 'still enjoy a generally high appreciation in the population', as Anton described. Compared to controlling and punishing institutions, such as the police, they are more appreciated. Many shared, however, incidents in which patients, relatives or other third parties directed physical or verbal violence against them or co-workers. Violence and threats were a big concern in the field. Some said incidents increased, an observation that research seems to support (Dressler, 2017; Lindner, 2022). For example, Lindner (2022, pp 13–14) assumes that increasing ED utilisation, situational crowding, and associated wait times have contributed to frustration and incidents between patients and providers.

More frequent than overt threats and violence was, however, the devaluation that providers observed. As Mr Leidner explained, the EMS and fire brigade 'slipped down in the valuation of the citizens'. People would see them as a 'contact point for everything where I'm at a loss'. He continued, 'People no longer take the trouble to look: "Wait, the fire brigade is the emergency medical service, after all, so when it comes to life-threatening things."' The rising demands and the violation of the illusio led many to reconsider their continued work in the field, as the next section will demonstrate.

Disengaging or finding a niche: providers' ways of coping

While for many doctors, the ED is an obligatory part of their training and thus a 'transit station', for many nurses and EMS workers, it represented an 'end to a long journey'. For example, for nurses, EDs appeared more attractive than working in stations as they included less heavy lifting, greater variety of cases, and flatter working hierarchies, as some explained. These aspects motivated nurse Astrid (with around 30 years of work experience) and nurse Kevin (with less than 10 years of experience) to change from station-based work to the ED. Also, higher-trained EMS workers could work in EDs, and applied for positions.

Nurse manager Astrid explained she frequently received job applications from EMS workers for the nursing staff. Those applicants, she assumed, tried to 'make sure to feather their own nest as time comes'.[2] She explained as they aged, EMS workers were concerned about the increasing workloads, intensity, and heavy lifting in the EMS service; the conditions made some consider and apply for working in EDs. Bridging the discrepancy between competence and practice also influenced this step. EMS worker Nicole, who changed from the EMS service to working in the ED, explained her transition as based in professional interests. She wanted to gain insights into the clinical part of the work, and in *treating* patients, in contrast to simply monitoring and transporting them.

Within the ED, positions and options for career development particularly for non-doctoral providers were scarce. Some, such as Astrid, were experienced enough to move up the occupational hierarchy, becoming responsible for managing nursing staff. Others, such as nurse Christiane with around 15 years of experience, enrolled for a bachelor's degree in nursing management, qualifying to work as nurse manager or other administrative positions. While Kevin welcomed career opportunities for nurses like that, Astrid worried about who would continue to care for patients 'at their actual bedsides' in the future.[3] She observed how caring for patients became less and less attractive. She concluded younger colleagues were more interested in studying and did not want to work around the clock, on weekends and holidays; they had 'another understanding of work and leisure'. A divide appeared between those working part-time and as temporarily employed nurses and those working full-time as employed by the hospital.

Some nurses opted out, while staying in the field, by increasing their autonomy. They worked as temporarily employed, meaning they contracted with a company that then temporarily sub-contracted with hospitals. Riedlinger et al (2020) refer to this practice as a 'silent protest'. It was a way for nurses to influence their working conditions by choosing and alternating shifts in specific hospitals and stations[4] and regulating their work time. Samuel with around 15 years of experience worked as a temporary worker and part-time. These options were 'ideal', he said. He earned 'enough to live' and still had time to follow other interests.

Experienced nurses like as Astrid considered, however, 'opting out'. She imagined opening a shop, considering leaving the field altogether, as it was not 'likely to get better'. She stayed, however, as she said to not have 'alternatives at hand so quickly'. For her co-workers she explained to be worried. She said:

> I'm worried about whether we'll manage to change the way the population thinks. Whether people will notice again: 'When am I an emergency, what is an emergency.' I think I'm afraid that the politicians won't manage to turn this around, that the emergency departments will continue to be overrun 24 hours a day, 365 days a year, by an increasing number of non-emergencies, and that the staff who works there will run the risk of resigning.

Many providers explained to be already resigned. Nurse Linda described undergoing a 'cool out': distancing from patients and her work. She would 'only do her job' and gave up her idealism to change working and care conditions for herself, patients, and her co-workers, she explained.

Similarly, EMS worker Philip said many of his co-workers were 'blunt' and 'disengaged'. He had applied for background duties, due to a decrease in his mental and physical health, as he explained and related to his many years at the frontlines: 'Meanwhile, I can say, "Okay, my time is up! Bones are broken, mudbug," but I'm here. I like the work I do here. I can look at things from a distance and say, "Thank goodness I don't have to do that anymore!"' Background service at stations was an option to opt out from frontline work that some took up. The disillusio seemed strongest for those at the lower frontline ranks such as EMS workers, nurses, but doctors experienced disengagement related to the patient increases and their mismatches as well.

It was not only low-acute cases that posed challenges – high-acute cases could also confront providers with experiences of disillusio. Anna had worked as a doctor in the ED and EMS. She recounted how she regularly resuscitated multiple patients in one shift, realising the cases she and her co-workers were 'craving for' were also 'emotionally exhaustive'. The work and experiences took their toll over their health, she explained. She wanted to make a change for herself. An ED manager recruited her to focus on low-acute patients.

Since focusing on these patients, her perceptions on them changed: 'The colleagues here always say, "They come with little things" and get annoyed because they want something real, but constipation can also be socially restrictive or restrictive at work. So, I see it differently now.' Although she also drew boundaries between (il)legitimate uses of EDs and 112 calls, she seemed to have found a niche within the transitioning field. Treating medically low-acute patients also was a niche for others.

In the EMS, experienced workers, such as William, found refuge in working with low-acute patients. His co-worker and supervisor Anton explained the 'young wilds' were motivated and liked working at the 'real' cases, supporting care for medical emergencies, while referring to responding to low-acute cases older colleagues would often say, ' "You know what? You can play the game without me. Then, I'd rather drive around in circles here all day and then I'm happy with it."'

During my fieldwork, I spoke with individuals who had moved or were planning to move to other hospitals, stations, districts, cities, or even into entirely different professional fields. To qualify for higher-level positions such as supervisors, managers, or planners, agents needed a university or college degree along with many years of experience or additional training. These qualifications were difficult for many to attain. Doctors were the professional sub-group that could exchange their cultural capital with other segments of the labour market with more ease.[5] Inside and outside career paths were diverse and secured their high professional and social status. Trainings for paramedics, emergency nurses, and nursing management introduced opportunities in which younger frontline workers engaged, while experienced frontline workers were more likely to stay in service and expressed a feeling of 'being stuck' (Margies, 2021, 2024) with their positions and the field changes.

Conclusion

Consolidating the wide access in emergency care had a downside for planners and decision-makers: both in EDs and the EMS, frontline workers observed resource scarcity and increasing job demand. The chapter stressed the symbolic side of the increases and mismatches and its effects on practitioners. Their field positions, habitus, and illusio clarified why some professional subgroups appeared more affected by the changes than others. The experience of an increased workload vis-à-vis an experienced reduction in practice autonomy appeared as devaluations and as endangering what practitioners identified with and stood for as 'helpers'. Autonomy reproduces the symbolic value and trust in practitioners as professionals (Hupe and Hill, 2007, p 282), in their formalised competencies and in the experiences they collect over years. Providers observed less recognition for them and more for patients. Planners, superiors and patients, it seemed, joined to break field promises of being cared for, trusted, and acknowledged as professional.

Researchers studying responses to change in organisations often assume homogenous responses among workers. More recently, research have shown that field positions and social positions influence how agents perceive of change and respond to it (McDonough and Polzer, 2012; Lockett et al, 2014). The chapter showed that although the increases and mismatches affected all, the change accumulated on certain professional and social groups.

The resistance to change showed how inertia to the changes needs to be understood in the context of symbolic resources as well as habitus and illusio (McDonough and Polzer, 2012; see also: Steensland, 2006, p 1283). Thus, frustration and resistance can be an expression of mourning the loss of resources, normalcies, and ways of 'being' and 'doing'.

Conclusion

Surveys consistently show that people call 112 and approach the emergency department (ED) for medically low-acute complaints (see Berchet, 2015; Coster et al, 2017). Health service researchers have studied the reasons for which patients use emergency care services functionally wrongly, arguing that low-acute patients exhaust scarce resources and thus endanger acutely and severely ill or injured patients while they could be served by ambulatory providers (see Lowthian et al, 2011; Booker et al, 2015). They also described emergency care providers' stress and frustration over the increased workload, and the challenge of managers to regulate the access to emergency care services (see Searle et al, 2015; Günther et al, 2017; Morley et al, 2018). Patient safety and work satisfaction are important and comprehensible research concerns. But I argued that there is a less understood symbolic side to the increase and constantly high patient numbers in emergency care, a share of which consisted of low-acuity cases. This side was my chosen focus for this study.

By focusing on the symbolic dimension of emergency care, this book shows that encounters between patients and ambulance crews involve more than a transport service. For patients, these moments often carry hopes of reassurance, support, and recognition within a complex and at times unresponsive healthcare system. For providers, they offer opportunities to fulfil professional purpose, gain recognition, and uphold a public mandate to save lives. The persistently high demand for emergency services has made access to both material and symbolic resources increasingly contested. For both patients and providers, these encounters are embedded in broader struggles over legitimacy, recognition, and value.

Drawing on Bourdieuan field theory, this book investigated the social causes and consequences of these developments. What symbolic gains and losses do the agents involved experience, both collectively and individually? I conceptualise these dynamics as a classificatory struggle: patients, as laypeople, and emergency professionals, as experts, compete over the definition of what constitutes an emergency and what justifies urgent care. Their respective positions within the social hierarchy of the field shape their capacity to influence these classifications and, consequently, access to care and symbolic recognition. The different capacities then encounter the inherent ambivalence of emergency care's dual nature: it is open to all, yet is designed to cater to cases of high medical acuity (Dodier and Camus, 1998). The increasing demand intensified the field's resource dilemma. Within this context, tensions emerged between key agents of the field: patients who call 112 and approach the ED, professionals at the service frontline, and the managers and planners overseeing the system.

To capture both the field's former social configuration, changes to it as well as its consequences, the book developed a theoretical framework based on the following social mechanisms and its attributes: *Relatedness*, *Embodiment*, and *Feel*. These concepts capture the agents' social positions, their embodied dispositions, their changes and challenges as well as the practical expressions of these. Situated within a historically informed perspective, this framework draws on broader literature on professionalism and the expert-lay divide (see Tilly, 1998, p 184; Luzio, 2006; Schinkel and Noordegraaf, 2011; Collyer, 2018).

From this perspective, the struggle over rising patient numbers and the share of low-acuity complaints is not simply a matter of workload or care efficiency and safety. It reflects deeper tensions within the healthcare field: shifting boundaries between laypeople and experts, questions of legitimacy and recognition, and challenges to trust. Understanding the hopes, concerns, and conflicts of both patients and providers illuminates these transformations and helps contextualise responses to them. It offers insight into the relational nature of healthcare with its changes, challenges, and the implications for policy interventions.

The book concludes by summarising the key empirical and conceptual findings turning to the individual agents and their collective positions, beginning with patients and then turning to providers and planners. It reflects on the strengths and limitations of the Bourdieusian approach in the context of this research and outlines directions for future study, along with implications for health policy.

The patients' perspective and the value of their mismatch to the field

Various factors mediated the symbolic losses and gains experienced by low-acute, mismatching patients in emergency care. Broadly, the institutional (doxic) structures of 'right' and 'wrong' pathways within the healthcare system shaped these symbolic dynamics through clinical protocols, narrow diagnostic categories, eligibility criteria, and the dispositional expectations and responsibilities of providers. Additional factors included: who the patients were (in terms of competencies, 'feel', and perceived social attributes); what they brought into the encounter (symptoms, reasons, expectations); and whom they met at which point in the 'chain of rescue' (including providers' sub-professions and value prioritisation). The following subsections discuss these findings in detail.

Patients' navigational sense in healthcare

The first empirical finding relates to the dimensions of who patients were and what they brought into the encounter. Low-acute, mismatching patients did not necessarily feel like they benefitted from the low-threshold access offered by emergency departments or EMS. Their perceived outcomes were shaped by expectations and needs that they brought along (also Afilalo et al, 2004, p 1308), themselves influenced by their social positions. I analysed patients' articulated expectations and related to social class, gender, migration context, and age. Rather than viewing these dimensions as isolated variables influencing healthcare-seeking behaviour, I followed scholars who conceptualise them as intersecting, collective experiences developed over life trajectories, informing perceived social position, expectations, and practices (see Bourdieu, 1990; Shim, 2014).

I used the example of patients who had already consulted at least one medical professional before calling 112 or presenting at the ED for the same issue – to illustrate a pattern in how people with low-acuity complaints navigate the healthcare system. I argued that this patient group is an example for a relevant but not well understood aspect that influences healthcare utilisation more broadly: the relational dimension of perceived outcomes from medical encounters. Their trajectories often began in ambulatory care, where they sought assessment, advice, or medication from GPs and sometimes specialists. These prior steps indicate a form of health literacy, in which patients functionally *correctly* match symptoms to medical settings. However, their paths often did not end there.

To understand this, I employed the concept of 'baggage' to refer to patients' accumulated medical and social histories (see Savage et al, 2015). These are embodied stocks of knowledge shaped by past experiences, which informed patients' 'feel for the game' (Bourdieu, 1990). Drawing on Bourdieu, I conceptualised *feel* as an anticipatory sense or 'investment sense' (Bourdieu, 1990, pp 66–67) that guides expectations and behaviour in uncertain encounters. It explains the shift from passive trust to more engaged, reflexive navigation (see Timmermans, 2020).

Many patients mobilised their feel to assess the trustworthiness of providers. In Goffmanian terms, patients evaluated providers' performance of expected 'normal conduct' (see Misztal, 2001) looking for cues of altruism, empathy, and professionalism. They paid attention to whether the provider listened, took time, conducted examinations, or displayed behaviours indicating competence. Trust was treated as a 'risky investment' (Luhmann, 1979, 24 in Luzio, 2006, p 553), given that diagnostic and treatment decisions influence access to resources and affect health outcomes. Patients, though dependent on professionals' goodwill (Luzio, 2006), were not passive recipients (Timmermans, 2020).

Different patients emphasised different indicators of professionalism, but common expectations emerged: time, conversation, understanding, and diagnostic testing. Patients hoped that exams and diagnostics in the ED would bring assurance, cure, and pain relief for sudden, enduring, or chronic illness.[1] I refer to Nettleton (2006) to interpret this as reflecting late-modern concerns with diagnosis and personal responsibility for health and risk management. Many patients were seeking not only medical assistance but symbolic recognition of their experienced urgency. Whether this urgency was acknowledged by providers – EMS workers, nurses, or doctors – was uncertain and contested.

In assessing whether a provider was responsive or unresponsive for the 'wrong' reasons, patients relied on their baggage of experience and *feel*. This aligns with Willis et al's (2016) concept of 'system knowledge' and Shim's (2010) 'cultural health capital' (CHC). While Willis et al (2016) highlight tacit knowledge of the healthcare system and its uneven distribution, Shim (2010) emphasises the differential ability to mobilise valued forms of cultural capital in medical encounters. My work links and expands on both, adding the importance of 'feel for the game(s)' – the ability to evaluate whether providers are acting with assumed 'good' professional intent: did a provider show understanding and appear to have the patient's best interest in mind or played a 'different game' (for example, focusing on saving time and other resources)? This suggest that patients evaluate providers based on expected and socially valued signs of professionalism in the medical field.

Patients drew on different resources – CHC, rhetoric, justification strategies, and a sense of entitlement – to subtly assert their needs.[2] Their feel and baggage help explain the socially unequal use and perceived outcomes of emergency care. Medical practices carry different meanings for different patients; outcomes of encounters were thus variably perceived. Patients with lower CHC and a baggage of negative experiences may have difficulties in developing trust in recommendations, treatments or diagnoses, and in generating a common understanding with providers, especially in time-scarce settings like EDs or ambulances (Shim, 2010, p 6).[3] Time-scarcity and brief encounters complicate communication with medical providers for patients with lower proficiency of German and lower CHC. Providers, in turn, may award, as Shim (2010, p 6) argued, those patients equipped with more CHC with more time, talk, and services.

The mobilisation of the 'feel' must also be understood in its historical context. Since the mid-20th century, patient activism and organisational reforms have redefined the patient-provider relationship (Shim, 2010; Timmermans and Oh, 2010; Willis et al, 2016; Timmermans, 2020). Movements for patient rights, especially those rooted in women's health, disability, and HIV/AIDS activism, challenged medical authority and emphasised patient autonomy (Timmermans, 2020, p 262; also Watkins-Hayes, 2019). Simultaneously, healthcare has become more standardised, managed, and commodified (Calnan, 2015, p 292; Timmermans and Oh, 2010). With all the stated benefits of such reforms, they also came with side effects such as a decline in professional autonomy and uncertainties in professions' value orientation, that is, the fundament of their legitimacy (Freidson, 2001; Luzio, 2006; Timmermans and Oh, 2010).

Governments and non-governmental organisations (NGOs) highlighted issues like malpractice and medical error, leading to institutional responses such as complaint systems and patient safety standards (see Luzio, 2006, p 559; Timmermans and Oh, 2010; Travaglia and Braithwaite, 2009). Patient safety standards, shared decision-making and patient-centred care became 21st-century healthcare policy goals (Stivers and Timmermans, 2020; Timmermans, 2020, p 262). Various healthcare-related agents advocated for patients' proactive health engagement, choice, and their position as informed 'consumers' (Allsop and Jones, 2008; Collyer et al, 2015). As Timmermans (2020, p 265) observed, 'patients are both more active in advocating for their health and have greater responsibility to advocate for health'.

My findings show that most low-acute patients were neither passive nor fatalistic. They asked questions, made requests, and occasionally even issued threats. At the same time, providers observed that their position had shifted – from 'professional helpers' to 'service providers'. Systemic access to emergency care alone did not dissolve the lay–expert divide or create encounters on equal footing. Patients' access to care remained largely dependent on providers' gatekeeping.

The symbolic value of patients with low acuity

The outcomes of mismatching patients' encounters, their symbolic losses and gains, were shaped not only by who they were and why they called 112 or presented to the ED, but also by whom they met in the course of care and by the provider's responsiveness to their needs. To examine how urgencies were acknowledged or devalued, this study followed patients' trajectories along the chain of rescue. It shows that patients encounter different frontline workers from different professions at different points in time, and that access to emergency care is processual and negotiated repeatedly rather than granted through a single interaction (see Strauss et al, 1982).

The timing and type of provider that patients encountered were crucial, as different providers, often coinciding with their position and their sub-profession, varied in their responsiveness to patients with low-acuity needs. Ambulance crews could decide on the hospital they drive to and whether a transport is issued; nurses could affect the access to the ED and processing of low-acute patients; doctors could decide on the diagnostics and on hospital admissions. Whether a patient's field-specific mismatched urgency was acknowledged or dismissed was not a given – it was negotiated within each encounter and shaped by the 'fluctuating economy' (Nurok and Henckes, 2009) of different logics in the field, that is, providers' situational discretion and value orientations in relation to their operational standards.

For many providers, low-acute patients were of lower professional value because they did not require the providers' specific emergency care training and competencies. They could also carry lower moral value if they appeared to be using emergency care for assumed illegitimate reasons such as convenience, potentially at the expense of others (also Wamsiedel, 2018). The low-threshold or 'wide' access to emergency care created a situational void for providers – what should be done when a person does not meet classificatory criteria for urgent care? Many filled this void with 'people work' (Seim, 2020, p 34), evaluating the social and moral value of the patient and their case. The labelling of such patients as 'garbage', 'misuse', 'trivia', or 'bullshit' reflected broader symbolic boundaries drawn between legitimate and illegitimate cases (also Jeffery, 1979; Palmer, 1983; Seim, 2020).

Providers often verbally or situationally devalued the more mundane health and social concerns for which patients sought their care, judging them to fall outside their professional remit. However, despite the use of terms like 'trivia', providers did not necessarily regard mismatching patients as fundamentally undeserving. In many instances, verbal boundary-drawing diverged from actual practice. Some mismatching patients received responsive care. This occurred for various reasons.

First, the reasons patients gave for accessing emergency services for low-acute complaints carried different symbolic value for providers. Certain patients and certain narratives could transform an 'institutional mismatch' into a 'moral match'. Providers judged these cases as legitimate and deserving (Wamsiedel, 2018). This was often due to providers' structural competencies (see Buchbinder, 2017; Metzl and Hansen, 2014). Many were aware of barriers to access other forms of help (also Vassy, 2001; Buchbinder, 2017; Wamsiedel, 2018).

Providers do not only treat physical and psychological complaints – they also witness the social conditions underlying health issues when entering patients' homes or listening to their stories. These interactions shaped providers' perspectives. This affected their perspective and 'social diagnoses' (Brown et al, 2011) on their patients' calls and presentations; it also affected their gatekeeping practice. I argue that this goes beyond explanations rooted in individual deservingness (see Lipsky, 2010; Lara-Millán, 2014; Jensen and Petersen, 2017; Seim, 2020). Building on research showing that providers' use of discretion reflects societal norms and judgements of patients' moral value (for example, Maynard-Moody and Musheno, 2003), I found that providers also evaluated the patients' 'social context', that is, their families, neighbourhood, bystanders, but also their own context, consisting of organisational peers and supervisors. Here, the provider's professional habitus and *feel* for when their professionalism was affirmed or violated proved central.

Second, discretionary decisions were not always directed for or against individual patients. Providers also used discretion in ways that reflected broader efforts at positioning themselves within the field: toward or against colleagues, supervisors, institutions, and external pressures. Emergency care is a contested field undergoing constant struggle over its organisation. In attempting to regulate access and service provision, providers engaged in relational work,[4] that is, distancing or aligning themselves with other actors (for example, hospital administration, the city senate), patients, and professional logics. In doing so, they sought to defend professional values, prevent symbolic losses, or claim symbolic profits.

In providers' accounts of their decisions, they often referenced logics external to their own profession, assigning responsibility to other agents such as ambulatory physicians, families, or society at large. When others were perceived to have failed in offering appropriate care or support, providers sometimes stepped in, providing a form of moral agency that Dodson (2009) calls the 'moral underground' of institutions: fulfilling responsibilities that lay beyond their official mandate. Moreover, many providers viewed external forces, for example, legalism, consumerism, commodification, and profit-driven management, as threats to their professional autonomy and symbolic integrity (see Noordegraaf, 2007). Some actively resisted these assumed influences.[5]

The study did not aim to identify 'good' practice in moral or normative terms. As Fassin (2008, p 263) reminds us: 'study[ing] [ethics] is not to presuppose its existence a priori and verify its realisation a posteriori, but to record and analyse how it is produced and justified in the course of action.' Nor do I argue that providers systematically circumvented rules or protocols. Rather, I examine gatekeeping as a symbolic struggle over professional legitimacy – how providers negotiated what was 'right', reproduced their sense of professionalism and public service, and influenced access to resources for themselves and for mismatching patients.

Providers presented as complex moral agents. They did not uniformly categorise mismatching patients as 'inappropriate' or 'undeserving'. At the same time, their ability to respond to mismatched expectations was limited. Patients' reasons for seeking emergency care carried different symbolic weights or what Dodier and Camus (1998, p 413) term 'mobilization worth'. But providers were not entirely autonomous agents. They were embedded in networks of interdependent accountabilities (see Hupe and Hill, 2007; Seim, 2020). Patients' needs and expectations sometimes exceeded the actions that providers could take at a given moment.

The next section now turns to the providers' perspective and explores the impact of high work demand due to patient numbers on providers' access to (symbolic) resources and how this was influenced by institutional responses.

The providers' perspective and their experienced loss of professionalism

Research on organisational change in healthcare often concentrates on its immediate, tangible effects, that is, how workers psychologically adapt to new roles and structures by rating their satisfaction or productivity, or how labour struggles emerge around conditions and pay (see, for example, Jacobs et al, 2013; Jacobsson et al, 2020; Seim, 2020). This book also traces such dynamics: experiences of increased workloads, stretched resources, overwork, fluctuating teams, retraining, and shifting responsibilities placed significant strain on providers and seemed to trigger direct responses: protests, sick leave, and boundary-setting.

But not all consequences of these changes seemed immediately apparent or intelligible. As well as physical exhaustion, struggles at work and sick leave, the symbolic foundation of professional practice appeared to be under pressure as well. The third empirical finding of this study therefore concerns the symbolic losses and gains experienced by providers amid increased and persistently high patient numbers. The analysis draws conceptually on hysteresis, disillusio, and professionalism as symbolic capital (see McDonough, 2006; Schinkel and Noordegraaf, 2011; McDonough and Polzer, 2012).

Hysteresis and disillusio at the emergency care service frontline

Profound and sudden changes within a field, as researchers have shown, make it difficult for some agents to develop corresponding practices and can result in hysteresis (McDonough, 2006; McDonough and Polzer, 2012; Margies, 2021, 2024). The habitus of frontline workers and their moments of hysteresis served as a seismograph for transformations in emergency care and in neighbouring fields, such as patients' fields, professional peers, and healthcare overall. Hysteresis refers to a temporal-cultural lag and maladaptation to a field (McDonough and Polzer, 2012, p 359). It can arise abruptly and have wide social repercussions; this book also shows that it can progress gradually and affect more narrowly defined social groups. This became evident in the rising and persistently high patient numbers in emergency care, as well as in the disproportionate impact on certain professional groups – particularly older, more experienced EMS workers and nurses – compared with others, such as younger paramedics and doctors who have recently entered the field.

Following McDonough (2006), I suggest that healthcare brings together diverse professions organised as a public service. I therefore employ the notion of a public service habitus (McDonough, 2006), a set of dispositions that links the various healthcare sub-professions. The public service habitus entails specific position-takings, such as loyalty to the public good, that are central to professionals' self-understanding and identity. Observing a declining capacity to fulfil these and the presumed causes of this decline violated what many providers expected to stand for and work toward. This finding shows that resistance to organisational change is not simply a reaction to new rules that appear to curb frontline workers' autonomy. Although labour struggles formed part of this resistance, the concepts of hysteresis and disillusio help to conceptualise these responses as violations of embodied, pre-reflexive beliefs in the field (McDonough, 2006).

The observed shifts challenged frontline workers' position as professionals in society and jeopardised the legitimacy of their profession itself – a painful experience that led some to disillusio and to disengagement within, or even withdrawal from, the field by finding a niche or leaving it altogether. Disillusio describes disengagement from the field and carries a social-inequality dimension. I showed that providers with lower (para)medical qualifications and greater age perceived fewer opportunities to change the field and therefore sought to adapt to the situation, contributing to scholarship on deprofessionalisation (Timmermans and Oh, 2010; Hupe, 2012; Betz and O'Connell, 2014).

The next subsection demonstrates that disengagement was aggravated by the observation that patients and superiors have increasingly failed to keep their field-specific promises of care and recognition.

Premises and promises of professionalism

Working as professional produced expectations about field positions and relations for providers in emergency care. Many expected trust and autonomy in fulfilling their work and mandate. They also expected care and support from their superiors, and recognition for their work from patients. These expectations concerned their access to symbolic capital or, more broadly, to 'professionalism' (Schinkel and Noordegraaf, 2011). These field promises appeared to be violated by the patient numbers, institutional responses to those, and the ways in which patients negotiated their encounters with providers.

Providers at the service frontline perceived these changes as driven by patients and external fields, and as mediated through their superiors and planners. Providers' social diagnoses of the patient increase and constantly high numbers, and their interpretations of the underlying causes highlight the ways in which they experienced a loss or decline in symbolic capital.[6]

Some providers experienced a loss in symbolic capital through devaluation and value deflation: first, they observed a shift in their relationship with superiors. It appeared to have changed from one of recognition and trust in their work to one of legalism and control (see Misztal, 2005, p 190). However, providers did not frame accountability measures as a general 'assault' on their practice (Lipsky, 2010, p 159) and thus as illegitimate. Many welcomed patient safety standards, particularly in light of high case numbers. They also acknowledged the legitimate authority of their superiors to establish such standards. Nonetheless, many criticised the extent to which these standards appeared to replace their former professional standing and years of experience. They questioned why their training and accumulated expertise seemed to have lost value.

From a conceptual perspective, providers observed a symbolic shift in their position; they observed a devaluation of their cultural capital and experience as well as a repositioning from a professional 'who knows what is best' for the patient to an ordinary worker and service provider who executes rules and protocols (discussed by scholars as proletarianisation and deprofessionalisation, see Timmermans and Oh, 2010, p S94). The experienced shift from 'professional' to 'service provider' is particularly impactful, given that healthcare professions are knowledge-based professions and have long been legitimately expected to 'know what is best' for the patient (see Luzio, 2006). Such perceptive schemata are deeply engrained into the professional being and part of collective and embodied histories (see McDonough, 2006; McDonough and Polzer, 2012).

Second, profession's monopoly on diagnostic means and health(care)-related knowledge has changed – and partly dissolved. While patients or laypeople long were neither in a position to make advanced health(care)-related assessments based on the lack of expertise and diagnostic means that professions had monopolised, patients now have access to vast information and digital diagnostic technology (Lupton, 2013; Lupton and Jutel, 2015). The 'engaged patient' (Timmermans, 2020) who has both the responsibility for their health and more information on it, challenges the authority and 'purity' of healthcare professions. The shifted position appeared for many as mediated by logics of other fields (for example, legal field, market) and their superiors as well as their superiors' superiors (for example, hospital managements). Professionalism in itself, as Schinkel and Noordegraaf (2011, p 67) argue is a symbolic resource based on exclusivity and scarcity. To providers, some patients appeared as experts of their own medical urgency, who were allowed to decide for themselves about their need for care and services. This undermined professional logics of expertise as providers were not expected to divert patients who they assessed as less medically acute.

For planners, the classificatory struggle between mismatching patients and providers resulted in a challenging mediator position. Their decisions regarding institutionalised rules and classifications not only established eligibility criteria for accessing medical services, but also generated symbolic value for some, while resulting in symbolic loss for others, in the form of diminished legitimacy, recognition, or devaluation.

Providers at times questioned the policy goals pursued by their superiors, planners and other decision-makers, thereby questioning their symbolic authority and legitimacy. Given that superiors and planners are positioned within fields shaped by accounting, epidemiology, public health, and the proliferation of standards aimed at enhancing patient safety and reducing legal liability (Heimer et al, 2005; Timmermans and Epstein, 2010), and in light of the current absence of clear standards and evidence for diverting low-acuity patients, planners and managers faced difficulties in diverting these patients.

Increasingly, however, research engages in developing standards and algorithms[7] aiming at safely assessing and redirecting low-acute patients to alternative ambulatory settings. These efforts may facilitate reconciliation of the relationship between superiors and providers and could also reshape the dynamic between providers and patients (see section 'From findings to future research and policy implications').

(Dis)advantages of using a Bourdieusian framework

This part describes how Bourdieu's field approach 'has been good to think with' (Lamont, 2012), and how it was not.

Starting with a drawback, Bourdieu was often charged for being too abstract and distanced to the everyday life (Back, 2015, p 14). Therefore, I included researchers who conducted qualitative and ethnographic work and who 'translated' the Bourdieusian approach and concepts. In respect to the structure–agency divide, Threadgold (2018) writes that scholars continue to relate Bourdieu to structural determinism. Instead, I followed the suggestions of scholars who emphasise the relationality (for example, symbolic capital, recognition, and symbolic violence) and agency (for example, feel for the game and illusio) of Bourdieusian concepts (Veenstra and Burnett, 2014; Silva, 2016; Wacquant, 2016; Threadgold, 2018).

Furthermore, Bourdieu's approach characterises agents as profit-maximising and self-interested actors, giving little room for moral agency and morality as an end in itself (Lamont, 1992, p 180). In response to this critique, I differentiated between primary and secondary habitus to account for the appeal and normative dimension of professions that 'do good'. With this, then, symbolic profits do not emerge from deliberate normative acts but as by-product of morally valued tasks.

Bourdieu's framework provided me with several advantages. The appeal of a Bourdieusian framework, as Emirbayer and Johnson (2008, p 5) write, lies in 'its ability to draw together ideas and insights that have already been explored by others … – but … within a more unitary, elegant, and encompassing framework of analysis'. I do not claim that the Bourdieusian framework serves as a blueprint for social life. Nevertheless, Bourdieu's approach is comprehensive and offers researchers a set of conceptual tools to think with. These tools, or conceptualisations of social mechanisms and attributes, enabled me to relate field dynamics and transformations to individuals' positions, their relationships with others, their immersion in a field, and their eventual disengagement from it.

Bourdieu's emphasis on the relational nature of social life aligned with the 'looping back' of field changes and their consequences that I had observed and set out to study. His framework helped me make conceptual sense of the collective histories of belief, dilemma, and expectation described by providers, planners and patients. Because Bourdieu's approach spans multiple analytical levels of social life, it allowed me to embed and contextualise present-day practices and subjectivities within the broader historical and ongoing professionalisation struggles. These struggles have (re)produced specific social arrangements and hierarchies in healthcare – arrangements that were increasingly challenged by the high patient numbers.

I expanded on Bourdieu by broadening the concept of patients' and providers' 'feel' in reference to the 'engaged patient' (Timmermans, 2020) and the 'fluctuating economy' (Nurok and Henckes, 2009) of emergency care service frontline work. It emphasised the different logics that shape patients' healthcare navigation and negotiation and providers' practices as they act within a field influenced by multiple others. The 'feel' helps patients like providers to assess the situation and prioritise accordingly. In doing so, patients and providers also contribute to the ongoing transformation of the healthcare field.

While Charles Tilly (1998) and Dorothy Smith (2005) would have provided a suitable conceptual framework for studying classificatory struggles around – and categorisation of urgency, the professional institution of emergency care and its low-threshold (yet stratified) access, and the reproduction of social hierarchies and inequalities in healthcare, I settled on the Bourdieusian field approach. I saw particular advantage in its emphasis on symbolic capital, the dialectic relation between embodiment skill and expectation (habitus) and healthcare arrangements (field), and the more or less direct struggles between agents both in concrete encounters and within the broader social hierarchies of social space.

From findings to future research and policy implications

While this study offers an operationalisation of emergency care for sociological analysis and a framework for understanding its challenges, it also has limitations and leaves several questions unanswered. Before turning to these in more detail, I briefly outline the main limitations.

First, the research was conducted during a period marked by intense public and organisational debate about crowding in EDs and the extensive use of EMS. Although such debates recur periodically, it is important to consider that this context may have significantly shaped perspectives – particularly those of providers. More recent research is therefore needed to assess whether the perceived distress associated with low-acute and mismatching patients persists in the field.

Second, the focus on low-acute cases may have downplayed the strain that high-acute patients also place on providers.

Third, analysing EDs and EMS as a single field may have downplayed the habitual – 'qualitative leap' (Bourdieu and Wacquant, 1992, p 104) – and organisational differences between them.

Fourth, the focus on EMS and EDs also neglected their broader organisational contexts, namely fire brigades and hospitals. These organisations operate according to their own logics and are themselves embedded in fields that shape their organisational contexts, including funding and standards for care provision.

Future research may address these limitations as well as the additional questions outlined below.

Future research agenda

The following section sets out these questions as a future research agenda.

The book described the presence of patient relatives, co-workers, institutional agents, and others who support healthcare decisions of patients in moments of need, but did not fully explore their importance. Other accompanying individuals often provide patients with system knowledge and CHC, and help to raise their visibility in healthcare settings. Research shows that the presence of, for example, family members and others influences if and how people get medical help (Pescosolido, 1992; Small and Sukhu, 2016; Dhand et al, 2019); they also show that such presence influences the interactional dynamic of medical encounters (Barone et al, 1999). Future research could improve our understanding of how people decide which medical help to approach, and how patients negotiate legitimacy in encounters by studying the relational dynamics of dyads turning into triads (see Barone et al, 1999).

Parts of the analysis focused on patients' trajectories. This perspective made it possible to show that factors such as temporal and sensorial normalcies, the professional value of a case, the social value of a patient, adherence to protocols and standards, professional ethics, and other elements may influence providers' (un)responsiveness with patients at various stages of the chain of rescue. However, I did not systematically examine individual providers' (un) responsiveness to patients in a *cross-sectional* manner. For instance, what role does a provider's professional status and their own social background play in shaping their encounter with specific patient groups, for example, in terms of social status or living circumstances, perceived gender, or ethnic background?

Research suggests frontline workers respond differently to different patients or clients (Maynard-Moody and Musheno, 2003; Watkins-Hayes, 2009; Maynard-Moody and Portillo, 2011). For example, Peck and Conner (2011) show that patients' perceived gendered and racial differences influence how cooperative and involving or authoritative doctors are in encounters. Wingfield (2019) shows that healthcare professionals of colour who work in resource scarce settings that serve to marginalised populations, engage in unpaid extra labour (termed 'equity work'), making healthcare services more accessible. An ethnographic approach would be needed that follows individual frontline workers for a longer period of time, study their encounters with different patients, get an in-depth understanding of their working contexts (for example, team dynamics, working hierarchies, department-structure, resource availability, setting-specific protocols) and systematically elaborate on how these individual aspects may influence each other how and when (potentially drawing on Nurok and Henckes's [2009] fluctuating economy).

An increasingly diverse workforce in healthcare leads to another research desiderate: studying patients' (dis)trust in providers and their perceived social background. Recent research shows, for example, that among patients who seek second opinions in medical care, male patients are more likely to seek a same-sex second opinion when a female medical doctor consulted with them first (de Vaan and Stuart, 2022). Also, this book and others focused largely on (dis)trust in medical doctors. Less is known about which aspects patients rely on with nurses, and EMS workers.

Another central – but neglected – perspective in this book is that of urban space. Lipsky (2010, p 28) suggested that the practices of street-level bureaucrats from the same agency may differ according to whether off-branch offices are located in a small and homogenous or large and heterogenous city. Atkinson (1995) shows, in a similar vein, how settings and medical work differs between places, directing attention to compositions, relations, and hierarchies within teams, differences in patient groups, and production of local routines and knowledges. I conducted research in different EDs and EMS stations but did not elaborate in detail on the role of place (for example, spatial stigma), specific work routines in settings and within teams – or the role of the department structure of hospitals. A systematic approach and long-term field stays in individual settings could add the layer of space, for example, inquire if specific reasons for approaching emergency care are more or less (il)legitimate in different urban areas and their medical settings.

Lastly, the field has begun to adapt institutionally in response to the high patient numbers and low-acuity patients. Future research should engage with the consequences of these measures, not only in terms of their effectiveness in reducing costs, facilitating workflow, and improving patient safety, but also in terms of their impact on providers' professional self-understanding, and on patients' healthcare navigation and experiences with these novel forms of care, for example, do patients perceive coordination and redirecting as responsiveness or rejection? Do such measures help to prevent conflicts between providers and patients, or do they instead create new tensions?

Policy implications of findings

As the number of low-acuity patients calling 112 and presenting to the ED remains high, policy makers and providers have made three suggestions on how to address the situation and improve conditions for patients and staff in emergency care. The following section summarises these suggestions and considers them in light of the main findings of the book.

Increase health literacy among the population

Scholars rightly argue that improving health literacy among the population is important for improving their ability to use healthcare and health-related information to their benefit, and for bridging the divide between laypeople and experts to some extent (see Schaeffer, Berens, Gille et al, 2021). But efforts to promote health literacy may have unintended adverse effects: specifically, health literacy promotion may reinforce existing social inequalities in cultural health capital and, as a result, exacerbate disparities in healthcare navigation and negotiation (Shim, 2010; Chinn, 2011). In other words, individuals who already possess higher levels of knowledge are more likely to quickly absorb, interpret, and apply publicly available information functionally rightly. Others, by contrast, may struggle to understand or effectively use such information, thereby deepening existing social divides. Further research into the effects of health literacy promotion, particularly with regard to the functionally *right* use of emergency care services, is needed. Complementarily, further research is needed on the extent and effects of providers' 'structural competency' (Metzl and Hansen, 2014) in encounters with patients who have lower health literacy and/or lower trust in medical practice.

In addition, my analysis showed that individuals who are seemingly equipped with health literacy do not necessarily make functionally 'correct' decisions or follow expected healthcare pathways. A sense of (dis)trust emerged as a crucial resource for navigating the healthcare system and provider encounters. Patients may also experience individual barriers when trying to access ambulatory forms of care, which makes it difficult to use services effectively. This suggests that efforts to improve health literacy must go hand in hand with a deeper understanding of third-party advice-giving, the structural and interpersonal barriers to other forms of care and support, and the processes through which individuals develop (dis)trust in specific providers, professional groups, and healthcare systems more broadly. It is essential to examine how these trust levels evolve over time and how they might be strengthened.[8]

Diversion of low-acuity patients

Alternative acute care settings located close to the ED or at the ED site, aim to divert and care for low-acuity patients more effectively. Current policy discussions and concepts suggest that these forms of care will be implemented and become increasingly important in the future of emergency care in Germany (see Bundesministerium für Gesundheit, 2025). However, the consequences for patients in terms of their care experience and their sense of trust in the care provided remain unclear. As the book showed, patients do not necessarily approach the ED or call 112 as a first step in their healthcare trajectory for complaints. Some have previously visited ambulatory care settings and developed a sense of not being taken seriously or a specific distrust toward a provider or their practice. These patients have been shown to call 112 or approach the ED in the hope of finally receiving responsive help, which may take the form of expected thorough diagnostics (for example, X-rays). As the consequences of implementing such policy changes for patients' care experiences are not yet known, patients' specific position as 'engaged' (see Timmermans, 2020) needs to be considered.

In contrast, providers may welcome the 're-purification' of EDs and EMS as it promises to reduce their workload in terms of care for low-acuity patients, reaffirm professional self-understanding and original mandate. Diversion strategies may enhance providers' confidence in planners' and policy makers' efforts to restore the doxic separation between the ambulatory and emergency healthcare sectors. These measures must be accompanied by research into the different positions to better understand their effects on different social agents and to facilitate mediation between the various positions.

Patient-centred care

Another policy suggestion complements the previous two, targeting the fragmentation of the German healthcare and social services systems. Rather than calling for behavioural change among patients, some policy makers and providers advocate changing the organising principles of EDs and EMS (Redelsteiner, 2018; Somasundaram et al, 2021). They argue that healthcare and social service provision has long been 'organization-centred' (following, for example, jurisdictions, narrow programmes) and should transform to be 'patient-centred' (following individual patients' needs, understanding their health 'holistically') (see Redelsteiner, 2018; also Krüger and Schuster, 2025).

A shift towards patient-centred care that facilitates access to health and social service may increase system responsiveness especially for marginalised patients and those with low degrees of 'system knowledge' (Willis et al, 2016). As researchers suggest, integrated and coordinated care can mediate social inequalities in navigating healthcare and social services (Reibling and Wendt, 2012; Schaeffer and Hämel, 2020). Such coordination risks, however, losing sight of – or responsibility – for the 'whole' person (Krüger and Schuster, 2025). Provision concepts would need to increase coordination among the different service providers for the individual patient and prevent 'shuffling' of responsibility (see Seim, 2017) between service providers.

Changing the institutional (doxic) arrangement and mandate of emergency care services (see Krüger and Schuster, 2025; Seim, 2017; Somasundaram et al, 2021) would challenge many professionals in terms of loss of professional capital, habitus, and illusio. Specifically, if providers attribute changes as external and illegitimate, resistance is likely to occur. In such cases, applied researchers suggest enhancing providers' capacity to influence the direction of responses to change or to expose both providers and superiors to their working logics and worries to potentially facilitate 'cognitive empathy' (Small and McCrory Calarco, 2022, p 20) and mutual trust in planning directions (see Hering and Beerlage, 2004; Smollan, 2013). When planning the transformation of institutional settings, consideration must be given to these relational aspects.

Appendix

Notes on methods and data

This book is based on my Sociology dissertation at Humboldt-Universität zu Berlin (supervised by Prof Dr Talja Blokland).[1] The following sections provide detailed insights into the formulation of the research idea, methods used, the data collection process, and the analytical approach.

This research was financially supported by a dissertation grant from the Heinrich Böll Foundation.

Formulation of a research idea

When I started my research in emergency care in 2018, I was not entirely new to it. Yet the choice to study the patient increase and their implications for emergency care followed a detour. In 2015, I conducted interviews with police officers, fire fighters, EMS workers, their supervisors and planners in two German mid-sized cities on the topic of safety planning and civic engagement (see Krüger et al, 2017). The semi-structured interviews were on safety topics, but interviewees repeatedly talked about increases of (mismatching) cases in the emergency medical services (EMS) service as a challenge to their work and professional self-understanding. Respondents who worked in the EMS also talked about their frequent contact with low-income and marginalised patients such as unhoused individuals and those who consume drugs and alcohol in public. These conversations tied in with my continuing research interests and laid the foundation for a research proposal.

In 2018, I started recruitment of field sites. The first interviews and conversations, combined with attendance of events and policy document research allowed me to map a wider field to explore and identify relevant actors (see Desmond, 2014, p 570). I started interviews with a Contracted Physicians' Association (CPA) representative, an emergency department (ED) manager, a district council and their healthcare planning unit. I wanted to get an understanding for the horizontal struggles between institutional actors first before identifying the limits or boundaries of the field. This way, I followed the suggestion by Collyer (2018, pp 121–2) to study the claims made and the positions taken by those who regulate the field, that is, identify major discourses and sites of tension. Question at that stage concerned: what is at stake in the struggle? How do social agents struggle – what kind of field-specific capital is used to exert influence?

Patient safety, costs, and funding, as well as numbers reported in policy reports and studies contained claims and served as symbolic capital for the interviewed actors. The interviews left unanswered what reasons low-acute patients gave for calling 112 and coming to the ED, how providers classified low-acuity in encounters, and what the increases meant for the access to symbolic resources and the intricate social web of the field. I then took the next step of talking to the agents who were mentioned prominently in the interviews.

I interviewed and observed service providers and patients, and settled on their perspectives and interactions as main focus to understand how they negotiated credibility and legitimacy in encounters. In addition, I continued conversations with managers and planners to contextualise conflicts within and between organisations and to examine processes of organisational adaptation. The analysis is structured along the following field positions within the 'chain of rescue': superiors (planners and managers), frontline service providers, and patients in EDs and the EMS. With that, I focused on the EMS and EDs each as 'field within a field' (that is, EMS as sub-field within the fire brigade; EDs as sub-field within the hospital) but did not conduct data explicitly on the perspective of hospital managements and the fire brigade. Scholars suggest studying at least two differently positioned and related agents when conducting qualitative–relational research (Blokland, 2012; Desmond, 2014, p 557).

The number of positions and perspectives chosen must be evaluated against the time and exposure needed to acquire what Small and McCrory Calarco (2022, p 20) call 'cognitive empathy' – 'or the degree to which the researcher came to understand those observed close to how they understand themselves'. The focus was chosen to ensure that the research addressed a research gap as well as data saturation regarding field changes, their social causes and consequences for planners, providers, and patients.

The next section provides an insight into the methods employed and the data collection process.

Methods and data collection process

I conducted qualitative data using the following methods or techniques: semi-structured interviews, participant observation in EDs, in EMS, and at events as well as policy document research to study the horizontal struggles between different agencies in Germany and *Urgencity*, specifically. The data served to map the field, its struggles patient numbers and low-acuity cases, and to ultimately understand their consequences for differently positioned agents in the field, their access to resources, and the relations among them. I got initial field access through one of the ED managers who offered to serve as a gatekeeper to his ED and further ones. My first explorative interview, alongside with participation in events on emergency care in Germany and *Urgencity*, confirmed that the risen patient numbers and low-acuity cases were perceived as a shared problem among EDs.

Table A.1: Overview of fieldwork and data

				Begin fieldwork	End fieldwork
1	**Interviews**				
	Professionals	Interviews	34	02/2018	05/2019
		Interviewed people	42		
		Average length of interviews	76 min		
	Patients in EDs	Interviews	66	02/2018	05/2019
		Average length of interviews	26 min		
2	**Participant observation**				
	EDs	Hours of observation	219	02/2018	11/2018
	EMS	Hours of observation	92	02/2019	04/2019

I applied for field access at two additional hospitals and, in parallel, within the EMS of *Urgencity*. Following invitations to present my project in the EDs and at the fire brigade and EMS planning office, I introduced the study to planners as well as to ED teams. After receiving their consent, I was granted permission to conduct further interviews and participant observation.

Talking to providers

I conducted 34 semi-structured interviews with superiors and providers in emergency care (Table A.1). I use pseudonyms for interviews, changed details of some interviewees (for example, gender, training backgrounds) to preserve anonymity. Some interviewees were specifically contacted according to specific topics, others were recommended to me by interviewees in a snowball-sampling fashion. I had a list of topics with questions that I wanted to cover in the conversation, even though I did not stick to a specific sequence and adapted the conversation if the interviewees suggested a direction in the interviews that allowed for a new angle on topics of interest. I did not aim at comparing the interviews along a fixed set questions but ensured that I covered certain topics of interest in each interview. I aimed at developing an understanding of the different positions, work processes, relations, and perspectives on field changes by involving different providers[2] (see Hammersley and Atkinson, 2010, p 117).

I adapted the interview guides for interviews in the EMS and ED as well as for the different operational levels (planning, management, and service provision). All guides contained the following dimensions: (1) personal background: questions on trajectories to – and experience in the organisation; (2) structure of the work: questions on how the work is formally organised; (3) field changes: questions on what changed in their work in the past years, assumed drivers for changes, consequences for changes, and responses to them organisationally, in teams, and individually; (4) intersection with other organisations (EMS – or hospital EDs) and changes to cooperation and work in the other organisation; (5) prospects of the field: providers' understanding of the field's future development. Additional to the interviews conducted in emergency care, I conducted semi-structured interviews with ambulatory doctors (n=3), of whom one was a CPA representative, a district council and their healthcare planner (n=1), nurses and social workers who provide healthcare for people without healthcare insurance (n=3). The interviews helped me to get an understanding of the field's working from a contrasting (partly: conflicting) perspective and thus served to triangulate the data (Hammersley and Atkinson, 2010, p 165; p 183). I identified conflict lines between the ambulatory field and hospitals, between the ambulatory field and the local political field, and between professional ethics and other accountabilities (for example, economic efficiency).

In total, I did research at three hospitals, which were differently organised as for-profit and non-profit, communal and charitable organisations. The hospitals differed in their size and share of patients who would access the hospital through the ED. I do not give details about the individual hospitals to preserve the interviewees' anonymity. This was an agreement that I found with hospital managers, staff, and administrations.

The administrations of all hospitals and the head of the medical and nursing staff in each ED gave their agreement to the study.[3] They were informed about the research approach, methods, and questions. I presented my project in ED teams during team meetings in which I asked for general verbal consent of the team before starting the data collection phase. I left consent forms as handouts. When conducting individual interviews and audiotaping them, I used written consent forms. The same procedure applies for the EMS. I interviewed staff in the EMS mostly individually, except for one group discussion. I drafted my project as a sociological interest in the reasons for the increases of low-acute patients and the consequences for the everyday work, provider–patient encounters as well as professional self-understanding in EDs and the EMS. In a similar way to the sampling of EDs, I did fieldwork in different EMS stations. Due to an offer in the field, I assembled a convenience sample, collecting data in four different stations.

My study design had the advantage of allowing me to confirm that the patient increase and its responses to it were not district- or setting-specific in *Urgencity*. And it allowed me to understand that the share of specific patient groups differed between sites. The study design had the disadvantage that I did not spend sufficient time in one setting to document patterns and variations in patient groups among the settings. Although providers talked about differences (for example, higher/lower share of older patients, higher/

lower share of patients without healthcare insurance, higher/lower share of unhoused patients) and I saw some differences between settings, I did not gather sufficient data to explain how these differences practically mattered differently in the different places or settings. This was mainly due to the limited time I could spend at each site. Therefore, the analysis refers to some place-related differences as reported and observed but is not intended as a comparison between spatial areas of *Urgencity*.

Talking to patients

I coordinated the semi-structured patient interviews with the staff in EDs. As a 'rule of thumb', as providers described to me, patients categorised as medically low-acute sat in waiting areas.[4] Doctors and nurses in EDs suggested low-acute patients whom I approached and asked for their interest and consent to participate in an interview. In some cases, I talked to patients and their relatives; in a few cases, I talked to relatives or other third parties who accompanied them (for example, work colleagues). In the latter cases, I talked with relatives about their expectations and their trajectory to the ED. The approach thus followed two selection strategies: (1) recommendation by ED staff, and (2) random and convenience sampling by approaching patients and asking them for interviews in the waiting room.[5]

The former strategy came with the advantage that I could directly relate both self-categorisation of urgency with that of professionals. Overall, I led 66 interviews with patients or relatives in EDs (those interviews vary in duration, ranging from 10 minutes to 75 min) – but divided into the three EDs, the number in each ED is too small and the sampling strategy was too specific to approach representativeness for a low-acute ED population. I did not sample according to specific categories or dimensions except for low-acuity; it does not allow for structured case comparisons along social categories or specific complaint categories. Also, I relied on providers' recommendation and thus reproduced their conception of low acuity.[6] My aim with the interviews was to explore reasons, expectations, and hopes people give – and what happens to the latter along their trajectories in the field. I asked patients for their reasons (noting several if given), expectations of treatment, regular source of healthcare and social care, if relevant to the interviewee's situation.

Prior to interviewing, I asked patients to talk next to the waiting room if the room was crowded to protect the privacy of the interviewees. I did not audio-record interviews with patients but took notes during conversations and completed notes after conversations. Approaching patients for interviews with a voice recorder felt obstructive. I worried that unfamiliarity of methodological traditions and techniques used in qualitative research and sociology would make me appear insensitive to patients (see also on the unfamiliarity between sociology and the field of medical care: Anspach and Mizrachi, 2006). I used written consent forms.[7] For patients (like providers and planners), rejection and stopping the interview was possible at any time. Some patients declined my interview request. I excluded some patients or withdrew my request when conversations in German or English were not possible. Similar to professionals, I used pseudonyms for patients and altered certain details (for example, their specific migration context or occupation) to preserve their anonymity when referring to their case in the text.

Participant observation in EDs, in the EMS and at events

In comparison to interviews with providers, participant observation allowed me to get more analytical depth, have non-directive conversation, and ask questions 'on the go', that is, when they came up in relation to specific cases, or practices of providers (Hammersley and Atkinson, 2010). Researchers rely on participant observation to document and understand the less visible and reflected sides of practices (Hammersley and Atkinson, 2010, p 3). A large difference to interviews is that practices relate to an embodied, immanent logic that is not necessarily 'articulable' (Koch et al, 2019, pp 7–8). While some practices are part of well-articulable routines, others emerge spontaneously (Koch et al, 2019, p 8). Participant observation of everyday contexts is thus an appropriate method to document and contextualise people's less reflective actions (Koch et al, 2019, p 8). I used participant observation: (1) during events on emergency care; (2) in EDs; and (3) in the EMS. I participated in four events on emergency medicine, in which patients increases were discussed either as the central issue or emerged as a side topic.

I made fieldnotes during stays in EDs and the EMS. I did not use tape-recording when in the field,[8] except for individual interviews with providers. During the ride-alongs with the EMS crews, I was sitting in the back of the ambulance vehicle. This is where the patients sit and are treated, and where the paramedical equipment is organised and stored. I largely accompanied low-acute ambulance operations. My focus on ride-alongs was the observation of encounters and reflecting on them with frontline workers. However, when patients started conversations with me and I had a chance to present myself and my project, I asked questions concerning their expectations in the ED or situation prior to calling 112.

In the EDs, I mainly observed intakes behind a registration desk, similar to the way other researchers conducted observations (Lara-Millán, 2014; Johannessen, 2018a). I took notes during the shift or made audio-recordings from observation. I transcribed and digitalised notes and recordings after the shifts. When doing fieldnotes, I focused on routines in the settings, actions, and conversation in encounters between providers and patients, as well as descriptions of atmospheres (for example, during overcrowding in EDs).

Doctors asked patients for consent when they invited me to join an encounter. To patients and new providers, I presented as a sociologist and researcher from university. In EDs, ED managers asked me to wear clothing of medical personnel for reasons of hygiene. I used a name tag that stated my name and university affiliation. During fieldwork in the EMS, I wore the clothing of crews and could not always present myself to patients. This aspect is problematic as the clothing might often have distorted patients' impression of my role in the field.

Despite applying methods typically used in ethnographic research, I do not claim to have done an ethnography. Atkinson (2017, p 2), refers to ethnography as a 'broad approach to exploration and analysis that is based on participant observation and the direct engagement of the researcher with the chosen research setting'. Ethnography entails the researcher's participation 'in people's daily lives for an extended period of time, watching what happens, listening to what is said, and/or asking questions through informal and formal interviews, collecting documents and artefacts' (Hammersley and Atkinson, 2010, p 3). An ethnography adds the factor of time. An ethnographic study, especially in the tradition of urban sociology or anthropology is based on long-term relations to field participants. I chose a multi-sited approach – both for theoretical reasons and that of practicality.[9] I borrow Atkinson's (2017) formulation of having 'thought ethnographically'. Thinking ethnographically involves contextualising social action and using first-hand experiences through participating in the field while starting off with an theoretical idea that informs the fieldwork (Atkinson et al, 2007, pp 4–5; Atkinson 2017).

Coding and analysing the data

The logic of abduction informed the data analysis for the book. Abduction is one of three different ways to relate theory and data. While deduction means that a researcher reasons from general ideas to specific cases, and induction means that a researcher generalises from specific cases, abduction represents a 'middle way' (see Timmermans and Tavory, 2012; Atkinson, 2018). Abduction describes an iterative process of going back and forth between data and theory (Atkinson, 2018). For Atkinson (2018, p 416), abduction informed the grounded theory approach as developed by Glaser and Strauss. In his view, researchers would often misunderstand grounded theory as a purely inductive approach 'by which "theory" emerges from repeated close readings of the data' (Atkinson, 2017, p 1). Instead, Atkinson (2017, p 1) explains that researchers usually enter a field with a disciplinary perspective which they adapt as they proceed.

In qualitative research, as Hammersley and Atkinson (2010, p 158) write, the process of analysis already starts with the formulation of the research idea and design. The formulation of the research idea and design stipulated an iterative process, interrelating data collection and theorising – 'so that the analytic dialogue … [becomes] a thread through the trajectory [of a project]' (Atkinson, 2018, p 415). Qualitative researchers' task is to study 'how … people view the situations they face, how they regard one another, and also how they see themselves' (Atkinson, 2018, p 415). Such a task is necessarily explorative, as a researcher cannot anticipate the answer to these questions. In consequence, researchers usually refine or even transform initial research interests and questions in the course of their study (Hammersley and Atkinson, 2010, p 3). Exploration means, however, not that a research is directionless (Atkinson, 2017, p 3). Researchers bring (disciplinary) ideas to the field and constantly engage with them in an 'iterative process between data and ideas' (Atkinson, 2017, p 3). The categories that researchers ultimately use to interpret the data are both based on available (disciplinary) knowledge and 'generated out of the process of data analysis' (Hammersley and Atkinson, 2010, p 3).

My conceptual journey started with the Bourdieusian field approach with the beginning of (desktop) data collection and first interviews. Relying on desktop research of reports, documents, research articles, first interviews, and participation in conferences, I began with initial coding (see Table A.2). Przyborski and Wohlrab-Sahr's (2009) description of grounded theory influenced my coding strategy.

Following Anselm Strauss, Przyborski and Wohlrab-Sahr (2009, pp 209–11) differentiate between three phases of coding: (1) initial or 'open coding', (2) 'axial coding', and (3) 'selective coding'. In the first phase, I sequentially coded interviews and fieldnotes both according to the dimensions or topics discussed in the semi-structured interviews and according to the topics that emerged from conversations and observations. I coded the data in MAXQDA and used PowerPoint to order and assemble memos. Memo-writing, as Lofland and Lofland (1995, p 193) write, is 'the written-out counterparts or explanations and elaborations of the coding categories (that is, the labeled ideas)'.

Memos are conceptual in nature and tie together and cluster different parts of data (Miles and Huberman 1994, 72 in Lofland and Lofland 1995, 193). I used PowerPoint as it allowed me to develop an emerging cluster of topics or concepts by sequentially assembling slides and assemble ideas and data fragments within slides and topics. I complemented initial analyses with reading of studies and literature as relevant for my topic and integrated them into memos.

In later stages of fieldwork, I added further interviews and fieldnotes from my research stays in the EDs and the EMS; I added interviews with patients, and further actors that helped me to delineate the boundaries of my field. I transcribed all interviews myself to further my familiarisation with the interviews and observations and began with 'axial coding' in MAXQDA

Table A.2: Overview of steps of analysis

Time period	Steps	Programme and techniques	Output and topics	
2018–19	Initial and axial coding	MAXQDA (Version 2018)	Around 14,000 codes (manually coded)	– Agents, relations, stakes – Classification of patients – Reasons for increases – Provider – patient encounters – Changes to the field – Patients' organisation of HC
	Memo writing: concepts and categories	PowerPoint	216 slides (1–3 slides per category or concept)	– Relating first theoretical ideas with empirical data, for example concerning encounters, fields, professionalism
2020–21	First writing, conceptualisation of analysis and theory	Word, paper-based writing and visualisation	3 analytical parts identified	– Changes in the field – Patients' and FWs' mismatching understandings of urgency – FWs' loss of professionalism
2021	Re-writing and re-assembling of theory and analysis	Word, paper-based writing and visualisation	First draft of the thesis	– Submitted draft
2021–22	Selective coding and further analytical writing	MAXQDA, Word, paper-based writing and visualisation	Around 2,500 codes (~ 2,300 auto-coded, 200 manually coded)	– Relations between FW and planners – Relations between FW and patients – Loss of professionalism and niche-building
2022	Draft re-writing	Word, paper-based writing and visualisation	Second draft of the thesis	– Submitted thesis

Notes: 'HC' is a short form for healthcare. 'FW' is a short form for frontline worker.

(Przyborski and Wohlrab-Sahr, 2009, p 211): I compared codes, identified orders between and within categories and selected important concepts. At that stage, I began to write first texts to lay out analytical thoughts. I developed a preliminary heuristic and structure for my analysis.

I wrote a first draft for the thesis in 2021. The writing and feedback on it informed the last stage of analysis and resulted in re-writing the first draft. At that stage, I used selective coding in MAXQDA, mainly based on auto-coding for specific terms and topics. I focused now on the relations between frontline workers, planners, and patients as mutually influencing their access to resources, which means I relied on relational concepts such as recognition, devaluation, and trust, which added and tied together the former analytical parts that described how frontline workers and planners classified urgency, patients navigated and negotiated healthcare, and the field changed and partly adapted to the increases.

Position on – and in – the field

I have sought to make my methodological choices in a responsible manner. Nonetheless, ethical concerns and moments of discomfort in the field repeatedly challenged this intention. The following section outlines four central issues that emerged in the course of the research: (1) immersion and acceptance in the field; (2) consent to observations; (3) giving up control; and (4) pseudonymisation.

First, participative observation is a frequently used technique in organisational studies and organisational ethnography (Kühl et al, 2009; Seim, 2021). It differs from 'observant participation' by the degree of professional immersion into the field (Seim, 2021). A professional membership highly influences the immersion into an organisational field. I am a sociologist without a medical training. My position was marginal to the working processes in the field. Doctors, nurses, and EMS workers gave me on-the-job training to help with low-level duties, for example, to change the sheets on hospital beds or stretchers, help patients to the bathroom or transport them to other hospital wards, and to make small errands (for example, going to the laboratory to deliver blood or urine samples). Other than that, I attempted to learn the art of 'not being in the way' to not obstruct the working processes, while still identifying occasions to talk to staff during breaks or quiet moments.

ED staff and EMS crews largely welcomed me to their work and settings. The contested developments in the field facilitated the relation between respondents and me. Providers approached me with interest in the project and talked about their experiences; patients, too, rarely declined to talk about issues of medical care, reasons for ED attendance, and the obstacles they faced in getting other medical help. As Small (2013, 2017) concluded: it is often easier to confide in strangers than, for example, your supervisor or doctor if you think you will face social sanctions. But I also encountered people with reservations.

I agreed with two frontline workers to not include them into observations and fieldnotes. Some providers remained critical of me and my project; not my intentions per se, it seemed, but the methodology. In EDs, nurses or doctors asked what benefit observations of encounters and interviews with patients would make to their situation. One nurse that remained reluctant in talking to me once remarked during a busy shift: 'Everyone is rotating, but you stand there and observe.' Even trying to explain my methodological approach and the traditions on which it is based, it was not always possible to bridge the discrepancies between the medical and sociological field.

Second, during observations in the ED and during EMS ride-alongs, I conducted participant observations and wrote fieldnotes usually without explicit consent of patients.[10] Even if there is a long list of researchers working in this way, that is, observing encounters in medical settings without having explicit consent of patients (Atkinson, 1995; Fassin, 2008; Seim, 2020; Lara-Millán, 2021), it produced discomfort. Also, a research tradition is not an excuse to not reflect on such a discomfort.

I searched for orientation in terms of research ethics. The methodological considerations of (medical) sociologists (see Atkinson, 1995; Rhodes, 1995; Desmond, 2007; Seim, 2020; Lara-Millán, 2021) and recent methodological debates in sociology (see Hammersley, 2018; Lubet, 2018; Burawoy, 2019; Wacquant, 2002, 2005b) were valuable. Also, I discussed research ethics in several contexts: with providers in the field; with other PhD students at the department of Urban and Regional Sociology at HU Berlin as well as with other PhD students from the Heinrich Böll Foundation with whom I organised several workshops to discuss questions of research ethics from different disciplinary angles.[11] The issue of consent in observations remained, however, a conflictual issue for me – and, as I learnt, for other researchers who conducted participant observation in emergency care as well.[12]

Third, the fieldwork that I conducted meant that I had to give up a certain degree of control on what I will see, hear, smell, sense or, put simply, experience. This is not entirely unusual to qualitative research. Conducting fieldwork in sites trained for people's emergencies while not being trained for it, posed, however, a special challenge. I had the opportunity to leave sites and stop observation at any time; but in the beginning of fieldwork, I worried about the feasibility of my project. I struggled with fears of failure (see also Mattes and Dinkelaker, 2019). Not only had the field access been a process of demonstrating staying power where I, at times, doubted the practicalities of my approach, but I also encountered fears of having overestimated my own abilities of enduring other people's suffering. I emotionally resonated with patients and their sufferings that appeared to be clinically low-acute or mismatched the field. I embody the position of a layperson with whom these operations often resonated differently than with providers. I was not immersed into the normalcies of the field. Even though I focused on 'non-emergencies' in the study, many patients suffered from chronical diseases, anxiety, or neglect, even if institutionally categorised as medically low-acute case. Embodiment and emotions can be valuable as insight into the field (Desmond, 2007, p 284; Margies, 2021, 2024; see also Wacquant, 2005a). Resonating with patients and crews meant to situationally 'take their side' and empathise with their stories and justifications.

In my last shift in the field with the EMS, I accompanied a crew for the second day. The crew was utterly welcoming; I accompanied a night shift that they described as rather exceptional as it included an unusual variety of operations. During the shift, we discussed, and I felt, the resilience that lays in humouring and bonding in teams notwithstanding the stark cynicism it carried towards patients and their conditions, and that frontline workers recurrently warned me about – not to 'take it the wrong way' (that is, understanding it as a way of coping with work and emotional challenges).

Another way in which I resonated with the stories that frontline workers shared with me were anxiety and repulsion. Frontline workers vividly described cases that haunted them and that shocked me. Among other things, they described the sound of bodies hitting the ground, the smell of burned flesh, memories of bodies caught under a train. Frontline workers shared those memories, not so much, I assumed, with the intention to portray themselves as 'trauma junkies' (Palmer, 1983) or to teach me (as 'apprentice') a lesson but to give me an impression of the other side of their job, the value and hardship of their profession. The meaning of life rescue that permeated these stories emphasised the discrepancy to the many cases of low acuity that they handled.

Patients, too, shared stories of suffering, neglect, violence, and anxiety with me as well as of what appeared as 'rational considerations' (that is, visiting the ED to get timely treatment). Patients like frontline workers and planners presented the urgency of their practice – in a relational attempt and gift to invite me to understand the 'logics of their games'.[13]

The things that people say and the ways in which they say it are part of relational work (Tilly, 2004, 2006). I reflected on why people said what they said to me and what it could tell me about the classificatory struggle in the field but also about my position. Frontline workers and patients alike seemed to resonate with me as I represented an 'external figure' in whom they could confide and share frustration and worries. On whose side we are on often depends on decisions of where to focus our lenses on and is impacted by our positionalities (Lofland and Lofland, 1995; Anderson, 2002; Duneier, 2002; Newman, 2002). The strength of relational sociology is not to take sides but to embed agents in their multiple social layers or fields that influence their practice, and to relate the different perspectives and stories of responsibility, blame, and justification (see Desmond, 2014; see also Blokland 2012).

I used the pseudonym *Urgencity* for the city studied. The patient increase that providers and planners observed and documented for *Urgencity* are not city-specific. Scholars documented struggles within organisations or between occupational hierarchies as well as between frontline workers and patients in other contexts as well (Vassy, 2001; Fassin, 2008; Hillman, 2014; Lara-Millán, 2014; Johannessen, 2018a; Seim, 2020).

Overview of interviews with professionals and patients

Table A.3: Overview of interviews with professionals, patients, and their relatives as mentioned in the book

		Professionals			Patients and relatives	
		Planner	Manager	Provider	Patients	Relatives
Number of interviews		34			66	
Number of interviewed people		42			68	
Interview duration (in minutes)		78			27	
Number of participant observations		46			4[1]	
Total N		69			70	
Year	2018	68% (n=47)			74% (n=52)	
	2019	32% (n=22)			26% (n=18)	
Position		10% (n=7)	12% (n=8)	78% (n=54)	76% (n=53)	21% (n=15)
Age[2] (mean, in years)		41 (n=63)			49 (n=66)	
Gender[2] (reference: female)		32% (n=22)			57% (n=40)	
Transport by Ambulance (N=70)		//			17% (n=12)	
Accompanied to ED (N=69)		//			49% (n=34)	
Having a GP (N=61)		//			82% (n=50)	

[1] More encounters with patients were observed; the number of participant observations listed for patients refers to those included in the book.

[2] Age and gender attribution mostly based on author's interpretation; I changed gender attribution for some respondents to preserve their anonymity.

Table A.4: Social context of encounters with the ambulance crew and in the emergency department

	EMS (participatory observation)	**ED (interviews)**
Patient presenting alone	6	32
Patient and another person present	46	34
Family member	23	–
Professional agent	12	–
Co-worker	7	–
Neighbour	2	–
Passerby	2	–
Sum of observed encounters	52	–

Notes

Introduction

1 112 is the German emergency number to reach the emergency medical services.

2 As Legg et al (2022) suggest, the term 'low-acute' refers to lower medical acuity of symptoms.

3 Titles are translated from German to English.

4 This number refers only to patients who became inpatients, and does not represent the total number of patients who became inpatients or remained ambulatory (that is, who did not stay in hospital after their visit to the ED) (Berchet, 2015, p 10).

5 In the EMS and patient transport, numbers increased from 8.32 million to 12.73 million between 2005 and 2015 (Seeger, 2019, p 7).

6 This book is based on my dissertation. Parts of the introduction appeared in Krüger (2023). Please see the Appendix for more details.

7 The term (para)medical is a reminder that this book studies both medical and paramedical work; the latter is based on specific and often short-term training in first aid with the aim to 'supplement … the work of highly trained medical professionals' (Merriam-Webster, n.d.).

8 I use the terms 'frontline worker' and 'provider' interchangeably. The terms 'superior' and 'manager' refer to individuals in higher-ranking positions among providers in an emergency department, fire brigade and EMS station. 'Planners', by contrast, are individuals not involved in service provision but responsible for its planning, typically operating in organisational units separate from providers.

9 *Urgencity* is a pseudonym used to indicate a city where emergency care providers observe patients approaching their care for various urgencies.

10 The application of the Bourdieusian triad (field, habitus, and capital) resembles the operationalisation of healthcare in the micro-meso-macro model of health services research (Ansmann et al, 2019). It departs from this model, however, by not analytically separating levels of social life, instead demonstrating their interconnectedness and historicity (see doxa, disposition, illusion).

11 Bourdieu (2018b) conceives of society as 'social space', that is, as hierarchically arranged field of sub-fields. He writes: 'Social space, as an abstract space constituted by the ensemble of sub-spaces or fields (economic, intellectual, artistic, academic, bureaucratic, and so on) owing their structure to the unequal distribution of a particular species of capital, can be grasped as the form of the structure of the distribution of the various species of capital that function both as instruments and stakes of struggle in the different fields' (Bourdieu, 2018b, p 109).

12 In theoretical terms, Bourdieu defines a field as 'a network, or a configuration, of objective relations between positions' (Bourdieu and Wacquant, 1992, p 97).

13 'Depending on the field in which it functions', Bourdieu (1986, p 16) writes: 'capital can present itself in three fundamental guises: as economic capital, which is immediately and directly convertible into money and may be institutionalised in the form of property rights; as cultural capital, which is convertible, in certain conditions, into economic capital and may be institutionalized in the form of educational qualifications; and as social capital, made up of social obligations ("connections"), which is convertible, in certain conditions, into economic capital and may be institutionalized in the form of a title of nobility.'

[14] Schinkel and Noordegraaf (2011, pp 85–6) write that professions emerged as positioned next to the field of the state (with its state nobility) and market (with its bourgeoisie), each monopolising a specific capital: 'Where the remnants of nobility possessed social capital as symbolic capital, and where the upcoming bourgeoisie possessed economic capital, professionalism was a third way, a form of status or symbolic capital based on cultural capital' (Schinkel and Noordegraaf, 2011, pp 85–6).

[15] Bourdieu writes: 'We also have *trump cards* [emphasis in original], that is, master cards whose force varies depending on the game: just as the relative value of cards changes with each game, the hierarchy of the different species of capital (economic, social, cultural, symbolic) varies across the various fields. In other words, there are cards that are valid, efficacious in all fields – these are the fundamental species of capital – but their relative value as trump cards is determined by each field and even by the successive states of the same field' (Bourdieu and Wacquant, 1992, p 98).

[16] Bourdieu understood a field's structure, dynamic and struggles in terms of 'opposition' (for example, economic vis-à-vis cultural capital, heterodox vis-à-vis orthodox) (Wang, 2016, p 355).

[17] A field position relates to a field disposition; it may be understood as a specific and durable 'inclination' and is part of the habitus (Suderland, 2014a, p 73). According to Suderland (2014a, pp 73–4), Bourdieu frequently referred to disposition but did not precisely define it and its difference to habitus to which it is strongly related. Suderland (2014a, pp 73–4) suggests understanding it as 'inclination'.

[18] Bourdieu defines the habitus as '"a system of lasting, transposable dispositions" that integrates past experiences and "makes possible the achievement of infinitely diversified tasks, thanks to analogical transfers of schemes permitting the solution of similarly shaped problems" (Bourdieu 1977, p 82–83)' (Shim, 2010, p 3). The concept helps describing people's social position in relation to (homologous) capacities to act in different fields.

[19] Bourdieu (1990, p 57) writes: '[T]he habitus is what enables the institution to attain full realization: it is through the capacity for incorporation, which exploits the body's readiness to take seriously the performative magic of the social, that the king, the banker or the priest are hereditary monarchy, financial capitalism or the Church made flesh.'

[20] In drawing symbolic boundaries, as Lamont and Molnár (2002, p 168) write, agents can make symbolic and moral distinctions and express membership to a social group. When these distinctions are widely shared, they become a means to secure resources (for example, recognition, income) (Lamont and Molnár, 2002, pp 168–9).

[21] When referring to 'the state', I follow Bourdieu (1994, p 4) in understanding the state as a set of 'bureaucratic fields' which concentrate different forms of capital (that is, the capital of physical force, economic, cultural or informational capital, and symbolic capital). The concentration results in a state 'meta-capital' which gives the state the power over these forms of capital, over the 'rates of conversion' and a variety of sub-ordinated fields (Bourdieu, 1994). The political field or field of power is the 'space of play', as Bourdieu (1994, pp 4–5) writes, in which agents struggle over the state capital (Bourdieu, 1994). A hierarchical arrangement of fields in social space, with bureaucratic fields and fields of power positioned 'on top', interacting with sub-ordinated fields 'below' (for example, education, healthcare, military, family), gives the state the symbolic appearance of unity, as Bourdieu writes (see Bourdieu, 2014, p 166).

[22] Schinkel and Noordegraaf (2011, pp 85–6) write that professionals emerged as positioned next to the field of the state (with its state nobility) and market (with its bourgeoisie), each monopolising a specific capital: 'Where the remnants of nobility possessed social capital as symbolic capital, and where the upcoming bourgeoisie possessed economic capital, professionalism was a third way, a form of status or symbolic capital based on cultural capital.'

[23] Different capital distribution and positions of for example, heterodoxy and orthodoxy, of domination and subordination and the distances between positions, for example, reproduced by different sorts and amounts of capital produce struggles and dynamics in fields (Bourdieu and Wacquant, 1992, p 101). Bourdieu contrasted dynamic and changing fields in pluralist societies with a form of social organisation he called 'apparatus', that is, when the struggles and conflicts immanent to his conception of field cease and all field shifts result from top-down actions by dominant agents (Bourdieu and Wacquant, 1992, p 102).

[24] As Timmermans (2020, p 265) posits: '[Engaged patients] … are both more active in advocating for their health and have greater responsibility to advocate for health. That is, engaged patienthood is not just a random occurrence or a choice but the result of physicians, government agencies, and other stakeholders delegating health care decisions, health monitoring, and treatment regimens to patients and expecting patients to do their part. At the same time, patient engagement builds on decades of advocacy from various social health movements and other social forces subverting medical hegemony.'

[25] In light of the significant developments in healthcare that have occurred over the past few decades, Timmermans (2020, p 269) posits that patients have been: 'Less intimidated by white coats, they have become more assertive, even if they tend to eschew open conflict and instead subtly assert their preferences by reading up online, presenting their symptoms to steer an outcome, or volunteering candidate diagnoses.'

[26] With scarce resources at hand, frontline workers must decide 'who to assist and who merely to process through the system' (Maynard-Moody and Portillo, 2011, p 256; also Higashi et al, 2013). This is not least because flexibility and responsiveness undermine themselves. Lipsky (2010, p 99) writes if frontline workers employ responsiveness and flexibility too often, 'their capacity to respond flexibly would disappear'. In other words, '[t]he impulse to provide fully, openly, and responsively for citizens' service needs exists alongside the need to restrict, control, and rationalize service inadequacies or limitations' (Lipsky, 2010, p 191).

[27] I relate to responsiveness in two ways: as frontline workers' expressed patient orientation and as patients' assumption about how client-oriented a provider is. Researchers define 'responsiveness' as relating to the non-medical expectations that patients have about healthcare, providers, and systems, for example, respect (including aspects like dignity, autonomy, confidentiality, and communication) and client-orientation (including aspects like choice, waiting time for care, quality of care, and social support by providers) (Röttger et al, 2014, p 87). Röttger et al (2014) show for patients, responsiveness is the expectation of an empathetically rapport with the provider and having the perception that a provider helped them with having their best interest in mind. The notion of responsiveness differs from that of responsibility and accountability. I refer to Gregory (2003 in Hupe and Hill, 2007, p 286) in differentiating 'responsibility' as being normatively and morally framed, from 'accountability' as practised and determined by rules and protocols.

[28] Busse and Blümel (2014, p 24) write: '[O]ver four decades, SHI was gradually extended from 10% of the population in 1885 to 51% of the population in 1925. Later, in West Germany, this percentage rose to 88%, whereas in East Germany virtually 100% of the population was covered from 1949 onwards.' The expansion of insurance coverage meant an expansion of medical care as public service and medical associations receiving a public mandate that needed to be organised (see Busse and Blümel, 2014, p 26).

[29] In German: Gemeinsamer Bundesausschuss (G-BA)

[30] The organisations are the German Red Cross, Johanniter-Unfall-Hilfe, Malteser Hilfsdienst, and Arbeiter-Samariter Bund.

31 On-duty doctors are termed 'Bereitschaftsärztin/-arzt' in German; they take shifts in an on-duty practice ('Bereitschaftsdienstpraxis') when regular ambulatory practices are closed. In 2018, there were more than 650 on-duty practices in Germany (Augurzky et al, 2018, p 11).

32 This book is based on my dissertation. Some of the content has previously been published in Krüger (2023). Please see the Appendix for more details.

Chapter 1

1 Category, categorisation, and classification are related analytical terms. Classification is the making of classes, defining of attributes, similarities and differences among its members or the things that belong to a class (Jenkins, 2000, pp 7–8; also Bourdieu, 2018a, pp 6–8). A category (and its application: categorisation) is an 'organizing principle' (Harrits and Møller, 2011, p 229) that results from a classification (see Tyler, 2015, p 500).

Bourdieu (2018a, p 74) writes: 'What is at stake in the battle over classification is the production and imposition of the legitimate mode of representation of the social world, of the mode of representation of the social world able to impose its authority and thereby to guarantee its own verification.'

2 My own translation from German to English. See for example, Hamburg Rescue Service Act (HmbRDG), §2, Section 2; https://www.landesrecht-hamburg.de/bsha/document/jlr-RettDGHA2019pG1

3 Operational ranks in the EMS (from lowest to highest qualification): rescue paramedics, rescue assistants, paramedic, doctor; operational ranks in the ED (from lowest to highest qualification): nurse, resident doctor, attending doctor, chief doctor and ED manager (see Blümel et al, 2010).

4 Most frontline workers in the EMS entered the fire brigade after acquiring a craft apprenticeship, which was a basic requirement for the operational service. These trained skills as for example, car mechanic, cook, roofer, carpenter made agents eligible and, following Desmond (2006, 2007), also a fit for (and reproduced) the technical work and team culture at stations.

5 After three years of service, providers may be appointed as civil servant.

6 Priority key words in the EMS: omega, alpha, bravo, charlie, delta, echo.

7 The colour hierarchy, going from red to blue, reflects cultural conventions on symbolically expressing danger and urgency and conditioning awareness and responses with colours (Fine et al, 1998). Red and orange are the triage categories that signify the highest urgency for helpers and the highest danger to health for patients.

8 Critical conditions of patients are announced by ambulance crews via telephone before their arrival at the destined hospital so that the on-the-ground staff is prepared to take immediate care of the patient.

9 Mr Leidner referred to a 'cut in the finger', a common example in the field, to refer to the growing helplessness of patients.

10 As agencies with a state mandate, many frontline workers explained that it was their task to educate citizens. Similarly, Lipsky (2010, p 61) described that frontline workers teach clients their 'client role' during encounters, that is, implicitly exchange doxic understandings of what the field expects of patients and their behaviour.

11 The definition is also shared by the emergency care association DGINA (Deutsche Gesellschaft Interdisziplinäre Notfall- und Akutmedizin) (see Behringer et al, 2013, pp 625–6).

Chapter 2

1 Misztal (2015, p 191) writes: 'People's views and understandings of their world become more visible when confronted with something new, strange and unusual, and it is in the process of

such a confrontation, by defining who are "us" and who are "them", that the idea of what is "normal" is constructed and the notion's rationale and values behind it are exposed.'

2 Frontline workers regularly described the 'population' or 'society' as an entity by which 'the state' (as another entity) is confronted, drawing a symbolic boundary between state/society which is common among frontline workers (see also Maynard-Moody and Musheno, 2003, p 22).

3 A hospital nurse coordinator, during an emergency care symposium in November 2017.

4 A decline in social activities can have various reasons, one of which is a decline in physical abilities and confidence in people's bodies. On an emergency care symposium in 2018 in *Urgencity*, I followed a presentation by an ED doctor on older adults' health and health risks. He talked about the less-known 'fear of falling' that some older adults develop and that results in a further withdrawal from social activities and in social isolation which, in turn, worsens physical and mental health (see also Lach, 2005). Older patients who fell and thus contacted the EMS were frequent, as providers described. They described their interventions in such cases as 'quick help' or 'quick fixes' for older patients who often rejected a transport to the ED and wanted to stay at home.

5 Mr Diestel, around 90 years old, explained he was alone at home, after his wife was admitted to the hospital. His doctor said he had been to the ED regularly and sent home again in the past weeks. This time the doctor planned to admit him to help him organise nursing care.

6 Anna compared the work between the socially mixed inner-city district with an affluent, socially more homogenous districts and said that she was more likely to discharge an older patient with symptoms of diarrhoea back to their family in an inner-city hospital, where people with migration context resided, than in another part of the city, suggesting people with migration context tend to live in larger families or in proximity to family members who might feel obliged to support.

7 Planners base *Hilfsfristen* on medical standards and knowledge on the average time frame in which medical intervention and first aid can save a person's life or prevent further health damage.

8 The abbreviation 'intox' is administratively used and refers to a person with symptoms of alcohol or drug intoxication.

9 An emergency fax is the notification dispatchers in the rescue service's control centre send to the closest available crew and department, so the ambulance gets to the patient in due time.

10 In a statement of the Federal Association of Medical Directors of Rescue Services in Germany from 2015, the representative medical director recommended, 'At this point in time, the Federal Association of Medical Directors of Rescue Services advises against allowing EMS personnel to leave patients at the scene of an emergency based on their own decision. This recommendation serves patient safety and the protection of emergency personnel from legal consequences' (Bundesverbandes der Ärztlichen Leiter Rettungsdienst Deutschland [ÄRLD] e.V., 2015, p 1; own translation).

11 This follows the institutionalised cooperation between the EMS and EDs, that is, the chain of rescue. Planners and decision-makers implemented this cooperation to improve the medical provision for medical emergencies (Ahnefeld, 2003).

12 Some described the problem that patients differ in how they described symptoms and degrees of pain, 'downplaying' urgency or 'exaggerating' it.

13 Researchers show doctors, in the early stages of medical training, tend to run more tests and exams to be safe, even for assumably low-acute symptoms (Searle et al, 2015, p 312; Seeger, 2019, p 28).

[14] A report issued by the ZI – a research institute of a health insurance association – compared how doctors diagnosed ambulatory emergencies in the ED and the ambulatory, on-demand emergency service (Neubauer et al, 2016). The report showed doctors in the ED were more likely to issue diagnostic imaging in the ED for diagnosed backpain (36 per cent) than in ambulatory practice (6 per cent) (Neubauer et al, 2016, p 28), indicating patients are seen differently for the same symptoms. However, this is at least partly due to the differences in how these settings are equipped.

[15] According to §323c StGB, see Seeger (2019, 21).

[16] Increasing standardisation in medicine, as Timmermans and Kolker (2004, p 183) argue, represents a shift in the basis of medical knowledge and practice from pathophysiology (based on learning about illness through case-by-case comparison) to evidence-based medicine and epidemiology (based on learning about illness through statistics and population health, that is, evaluation of risks and likelihoods for the occurrence of illnesses). Evidence-based medicine and epidemiology aim to 'strengthen the scientific base of health care and determine the effectiveness of clinical interventions (Sackett et al, 1996)'. It also aims to decrease variations in practices and to increase the quality of care as well as to contain costs (Timmermans and Kolker, 2004, p 177).

[17] Ambulatory practices get reimbursed by health insurances according to budgets, which define and limit the volume of services they get reimbursed.

[18] Share of healthcare insured people in Germany who waited more than three weeks for a specialist appointment was 30 per cent in 2019 (Aerzteblatt.de, 2020). Researchers assume longer waiting times for specific examinations, longer waiting times in cities and metropolitan regions, and for SHI insured patients (Aerzteblatt.de, 2020).

[19] As hospitals can issue examinations like an Magnetic Resonance Imaging (MRI) or gastroscopy within hours or days for in-patients.

[20] In EDs or to EMS personnel, as their reasons for calling 112 or going to the ED, patients described that their GPs or specialists were closed, lacked timely appointments, or rejected seeing them.

[21] § 116a SGB V – Ambulatory Treatment by Hospitals in Case of Underprovision (Ambulante Behandlung durch Krankenhäuser bei Unterversorgung) (Dejure, 2022).

[22] See Seim (2020) for a conceptualisation of burden shuffling in the EMS.

[23] Nurses, such as Astrid, named the change or adjustment of catheters as a problem. Catheters need to be adjusted or changed regularly, Astrid explained, and nurses have the training and mandate to change them; ambulatory doctors would be able to do so too, but assistant personnel are not qualified and thus often referred patients to EDs.

[24] A 2018 report on emergency care conducted by the *SVR Gesundheit* (*Sachverständigenrat Gesundheit*) problematised the EMS in Germany not being part of the SGB V healthcare system planning and reimbursement. The *SVR Gesundheit* is a central expert committee, commissioned by the federal government, which reviews healthcare developments and recommends reforms. The authors assumed this EMS' position sets 'disincentives' to transport low-acute patients (SVR Gesundheit, 2018, p 594). If health insurance would reimburse operations that include a drive to the patient but do not involve a transport or further treatments, it would disincentivise doing so, as the SVR suggests (SVR Gesundheit, 2018, p 598).

[25] Doctors also described the opposite; in times of *angespannte Bettenlage* (tense hospital bed situation), they could not simply admit patients, and for example, had to engage in patient exchanges with stations or other hospitals, or, in other instances, sent patients home again when it appeared safe to do so.

26 Frontline workers explained the fee covers and often exceeds the costs produced, resulting in 'profit' for the agency.

27 Staff in EDs described that EDs are 'cost centres'.

28 Schinkel and Noordegraaf (2011, p 67) write: 'We regard professionalism as a form of symbolic capital, the substance of which is constantly at stake in power-driven contexts, both internally and externally. … Within each professional field, the legitimate substance of what it means to act in a "professional way" is constantly at stake.'

29 Mrs Hirschauer, around 80 years old, went to the ED for clarification of pain in her leg. She said she could have waited until the next day to go to an ambulatory doctor, but she worried she would not be able to do it because she was caring for her husband at home.

30 Ms Klüver described how social mechanisms of reciprocity between neighbours complicated the exchange of support within her residency.

Chapter 3

1 I did not measure health literacy or other forms of cultural health capital (CHC) of interviewees in a standardised manner, in relation to the existing operationalisation. The different rating was based on the aspects that patients mobilised in the medical encounter. While Ms Wilke explicitly referenced her highest vocational degree and other pertinent details related to her medical profession, she provided sufficient justification for categorising her in a higher profile. In contrast, Ms Schwartz was categorised as in a lower profile, utilising popular media such as a popular television programme and a family member as sources of credited information.

2 For reasons of anonymity, the actual profession is not identified. It requires a moderate level of training.

3 Further examples included interviews with Ms Charon, Ms Dulek, and Ms Hoffmann: Ms Charon, a patient in her 30s, came to the ED for breathing difficulties that have lasted for three weeks. Before she came to the ED, she went to a specialist, but that one was so 'fast that she had not much trust' and she 'did not feel like the doctor was listening to her'. She went to another specialist who had ruled out a bronchitis which appeared 'more trustworthy' to her, but she still felt like she 'was missing something'. She wanted to rule out that it is not 'something worse' and came to the ED. Ms Dulek, in her 20s, explained that she does not trust her GP anymore because she 'doesn't find anything' in regard to her enduring stomach pain; she called 112 and came to the ED after her stomach pain worsened overnight, hoping for more diagnostics in the ED. Ms Hoffmann, a nurse in her 30s, explained that she had the feeling that 'doctors hardly talk to you' and 'don't really get to the bottom of things'. She continued explaining: 'They [the doctors] take maybe five minutes time for you and then you are alone with this again.'

4 Ms Gussew went to her GP earlier, but the practice was closed.

5 Thirty-four out of 66 patients from my interview sample in EDs were accompanied by a relative, institutional agent, neighbour, or friend. In my observation of EMS operations, in 46 cases another person (for example, a passerby or relative) was present; in 6 cases, the patient was alone (see Appendix – Table A.4).

6 The aspect refers to the patients' perspective.

Chapter 4

1 The telephone on-call service of Statutory Health Insurance (SHI) doctors.

2 As Maynard-Moody and Portillo (2011, p 266) write, 'Discretion – and its potential abuse – is important not because of its frequency, but because it is available to street-level workers when they choose to exercise it (Skolnick and Fyfe, 1993, 120).'

[3] In other cases, frontline workers made assumptions about the urgency of patients based on their presumed membership of certain social groups. This was observed in an encounter with a Syrian refugee (in a refugee shelter) in which the EMS worker responded harshly to the patient, assuming his expressed level of pain was based on 'weltschmerz' rather than objectifiable symptoms, or when an EMS worker did not take vital signs from a homeless patient, assuming a medically low-acuity case. Such categorisations risk prioritising patients' social 'frames', culturalising expressions of pain or other symptoms, which can lead to undertreatment, as researchers have shown (Holmes, 2007, 2013; Lara-Millán, 2014). In both cases, however, the patients were transported to the ED.

[4] Pain above 7 equates 'strong pain' and is categorised as the most urgent category ('orange'); pain between 5 and 7 is categorised as 'yellow'; pain between 1 and 4 is categorised as 'green'; see Timm (2018).

[5] With some experience, nurse Astrid said, 'You can assess this quite well. Who is the malingerer here and has perhaps already come through quite well with the number [the strategy of expressing a high level of pain] … and who is now really pain-ridden.'

[6] Frontline workers also talked about the risks of 'putting people into boxes', as Dr Lindemann termed it. That risk was present for nurses when triaging and for doctors when diagnosing.

Chapter 5

[1] Providers recommended some patients as 'typical patients' to me for interviews. As laid out in the Appendix, I did so when patients accepted.

[2] Hospital beds are a scarce resource, and doctors in EDs described the time spent on finding a bed in hospital departments for their in-patients; the availability of beds could inform doctors' discretion in admitting patients.

[3] These limitations have resemblance with the aspects Seim (2017, 2020) terms 'vertical forces'. Vertical forces are those of the capitalist market and bureaucratic state which influence the on-the-ground working through logics of, for example, efficiency and public accountability.

Chapter 6

[1] Chronic illnesses, high age, psychiatric diagnoses, drug or alcohol dependency, recurrent 112 calls by bystanders for homeless individuals and domestic violence can be involved when patients regularly use emergency care services (see Booker et al, 2015; Breuer et al, 2020).

[2] Parts of this quote have been published before in Krüger (2024).

[3] This quote was incorrectly attributed to another interviewee in previous publications.

[4] The form and content of emergency care reforms are the subject of ongoing debate (see Sefrin, 2025).

[5] Note that a similar overlap between (para)medical training and training in public health exists for scholars who work on – and argue for a shift towards social emergency care (see Fahimi and Goldfrank, 2019).

[6] A model that challenges the compartmentalisation of the body, psyche, and the social (Brady, 2012).

Chapter 7

[1] Due to the pseudonymisation, no further details are provided.

[2] In *Urgencity*, nursing staff from hospitals started protesting in 2020; the pandemic intensified resource scarcity and work demands for medical personnel. One main demand of the protests was more personnel. Doctors in German municipal hospitals went on

collective strike in 2022, protesting the violations against work time regulation and inadequate staffing.

3 Frontline workers in the fire brigade could apply for relocation to, for example, be closer to their homes or change teams. Not all applications were successful as some said, describing frustration with their lack of autonomy.

4 High workloads coincided with the stresses of working in shift systems. Kevin and Anna, like frontline workers in the EMS, explained how working in the shift system, working on weekends, and the demand for flexibility and to work overtime as a result of tense personnel situations affected their health and well-being and their private lives, as they had less time for, say, workouts, hobbies, family, and friends. Philip said he and his colleagues get 'burned' (*verheizt*), not having enough time to compensate for the stresses of work.

5 It accounted for new standards in emergency care and equipment and aimed at reducing the time until medical intervention reached patients, increasing patient safety, and relieving overburdened emergency doctors in the EMS. In response, *Urgencity* adapted and updated its EMS act. Central was the implementation of the paramedic act and regulating the replacement of the lower EMS training with the training as a paramedic.

Chapter 8

1 'Shock room' is a term for a room within EDs in which severely ill and injured patients are provided with first aid.

2 She used a German saying: 'Seine Schäfchen ins Trockene bringen.'

3 Hospitals increasingly fill 'personnel gaps' by employing so-called nurse assistants. Hospitals and other companies recruit nurse assistants from other countries (for example, people from Southeast Asian and Eastern European countries). A nurse manager explained to me how she would like to employ nurse assistants in her ED to help with cleaning patients, replenishing stocks, and so on. This recruiting practice increases the number of low social and occupational positions in EDs and hospital stations.

4 For Astrid, who as responsible for the staff schedule, temporary workers helped 'filling the gaps' but meant less planning reliability and stipulated the fear that co-workers might follow the same path.

5 Within the hospital, doctors could qualify as, for example, chief doctor, managing a station or ED. Doctors could also qualify as specialist to open a practice, or change careers to work in, for example, consulting, policy making (see Hanke, 2021).

Conclusion

1 Patients' expectation of evidence-producing tests might have, paradoxically, become an anticipation for medical practice during a time when practitioners debated the benefits of narrative medicine over technical- and pharmaceutical-based practice in ambulatory care (Kalitzkus et al, 2009; Struzik et al, 2018).

2 There were, however, also reports by providers and researchers on overt conflicts, verbal and physical aggression exerted by patients or their relatives (see Karutz, 2014; Dressler, 2017; Lindner, 2022).

3 Trust may contribute to adherence to advice and medication plans with potential positive effects for health and well-being (Shim, 2010, p 12; Zussman, 2010, p 1338; Nettleton et al, 2013); it can also have negative consequences for patients and their health, leading to overtreatment or undertreatment without the patient being aware of it (Shim, 2010, p 12; Zussman, 2010, p 1338; Nettleton et al, 2013).

4 Zelizer (2012) coined the notion of 'relational work' and based her thinking in the work of Charles Tilly. See Schilling (2019, 2023) for a study that relies on Viviana Zelizer's work. I use the notion of relational work here to indicate that people actively (though

not necessarily reflexive) manage social relations by distancing, boundary drawing, and by associating themselves with people or logics. This understanding aligns with the Bourdieusian notion of 'position-taking'. With the notion, I aim to account for the historic-collective and individual emergence of standpoints towards others (Emirbayer and Johnson, 2008, p 14).

5 For example, Dr Meinhard used positive discretion for Mr Müller, classifying him as deserving and classifying health insurance companies as external to medical practice, and changes in societies as shifting the institutional responsibilities for which no other actor accounted for.

6 I understand symbolic capital as an added value to the fundamental forms of capital (Rehbein and Saalmann, 2014, p 138) – in other words, as a form of (mis)recognition of legitimacy, status, and authority (Bourdieu, 1986, p 138).

7 See, for example, projects on an algorithm to standardise the initial assessment of medical urgency at the ED registration desk and the 116 117 emergency hotline 'SmED' (Strukturierte medizinische Ersteinschätzung in Deutschland) at the ZI (Zentralinstitut für die kassenärztliche Versorgung in der Bundesrepublik Deutschland, 2022).

8 For example, scholars assume that patients' lack of participation in healthcare planning and policy affects their trust in healthcare systems negatively (Wendt, 2003, 2007). Germany is an example of a healthcare system in which patients only participate marginally (with no voting right in the central decision-making council, G-BA). Studies may engage with the effects of participation in healthcare planning on more sustainable use of services.

Appendix

1 As part of the PhD process, the original thesis has been submitted to the university library (Krüger, 2023).

2 Along the axes of the organisational membership (ED, EMS) and position within an organisation (planning, management; frontline provision).

3 Due to shift changes or vacations, I had to re-represent myself and project in the field several times to individual frontline workers in the ED who were not part of the team meetings in which my project was presented, and I asked consent.

4 Providers also used the triage categories to evaluate the medical acuity of patients. They considered patients with categories blue, green, and in some cases, yellow as clinically low-acute.

5 This selection process followed the example of other researchers in the field (see Scherer et al, 2017; Schmiedhofer et al, 2017).

6 In four cases, nurses or doctors recommended patients for interviews who were triaged as low-acute first but were admitted as inpatients after doctoral consultation; I excluded them from the interview sample as the focus of the study is on institutional mismatches, that is, those patients eligible for ambulatory care.

7 Complying with the General Data Protection Regulation (GDPR; German: DSGVO).

8 ED and EMS managers asked me not to use tape recorders for reasons of data protection. This met my reservations of using a recorder in these settings as well, because, first, the short field stays where I accompanied crews for not more than two shifts made it unlikely to develop misrecognition of the device and trust in my uses of recorded voices (see also Desmond, 2007, p 287). I did re-visits in EDs that produced mutual familiarity in teams but continued to rely on making fieldnotes. Conversations with staff in EDs were usually brief enough to capture them in fieldnotes.

9 To not obstruct the working processes, ED managers and station managers gave me specific time periods for participant observations. ED teams usually hosted one to several interns

in nursing, paramedicine, or medicine. I was given access in weeks in which the teams had time for a field novice and her questions.

10 I used written consent forms when doing interviews.

11 According to the statute of the ethics committee of the Faculty of Humanities and Social Sciences at HU Berlin, the main supervisor of a PhD project observes the compliance with research ethics (Faculty of Humanities and Social Sciences, 2018).

12 I contacted other (medical) sociologists to engage in exchanges on methodological issues and practices. There seems to be a consensus on the fact that it is acceptable to observe interactions between patients and providers without gaining patients' consent. Consent is needed, however, when conducting interviews.

13 Bourdieu (1990, p 82) writes: 'Urgency, which is rightly seen as one of the essential properties of practice, is the product of playing in the game and the presence in the future that it implies. One only has to stand outside the game, as the observer does, in order to sweep away the urgency, the appeals, the threats, the steps to be taken, which make up the real, really lived-in, world.'

References

Acosta, K.L. (2021). *Queer Stepfamilies: The Path to Social and Legal Recognition.* NYU Press.

Aerzteblatt.de (2020). *Wartezeit auf Facharzttermin im Schnitt mehr als drei Wochen.* https://www.aerzteblatt.de/nachrichten/108921/Wartezeit-auf-Facharzttermin-im-Schnitt-mehr-als-drei-Wochen

Afilalo, J., Marinovich, A., Afilalo, M., Colacone, A., Léger, R., Unger, B., and Giguère, C. (2004). Nonurgent Emergency Department Patient Characteristics and Barriers to Primary Care. *Academic Emergency Medicine, 11*(12), 1302–10. https://doi.org/10.1197/j.aem.2004.08.032

Ahnefeld, F.W. (2003). Die Rettungskette: Eine Idee wurde Wirklichkeit. *Notfall & Rettungsmedizin, 6*(7), 520–25. https://doi.org/10.1007/s10049-003-0595-9

Allsop, J., and Jones, K.L. (2008). Withering the Citizen, Managing the Consumer: Complaints in Healthcare Settings. *Social Policy and Society,* 7(2), 233–244.

Anderson, E. (2002). The Ideologically Driven Critique. *American Journal of Sociology, 107*(6), 1533–50. https://doi.org/10.1086/342772

Andrew, E., Nehme, Z., Cameron, P., and Smith, K. (2020). Drivers of Increasing Emergency Ambulance Demand. *Prehospital Emergency Care, 24*(3), 385–93. https://doi.org/10.1080/10903127.2019.1635670

Ansmann, L., Baumann, W., Gostomzyk, J., Götz, K., Hahn, U., Pfaff, H., Rölker-Denker, L., and Nöst, S. (2019). DNVF-Memorandum III – Methoden für die Versorgungsforschung, Teil 4 – Konzept und Methoden der organisationsbezogenen Versorgungsforschung. Kapitel 1 – Definition und Konzept der organisationsbezogenen Versorgungsforschung [DNVF-Memorandum III – Methods For Health Services Research, Part 4 – Concept and Methods For Organizational Health Services Research. Chapter 1 – Definition and Concept of Organizational Health Services Research]. *Gesundheitswesen, 81*(03), e64–e71. https://doi.org/10.1055/a-0862-0527

Anspach, R.R., and Mizrachi, N. (2006). The Field Worker's Fields: Ethics, Ethnography and Medical Sociology. *Sociology of Health & Illness, 28*(6), 713–31.

Arntz, H.R., and Poloczek, S. (2012). Wann sollte man den Rettungsdienst nicht alarmieren? *Notfall + Rettungsmedizin, 15*(8), 661–6. https://doi.org/10.1007/s10049-011-1542-9

Atkinson, P. (1995). *Medical Talk and Medical Work: The Liturgy of the Clinic.* Sage.

Atkinson, P. (2017). *Thinking Ethnographically*. Sage.

Atkinson, P. (2018). The Spirit of Abduction. *Contemporary Sociology*, *47*(4), 415–17. https://doi.org/10.1177/0094306118779812b

Atkinson, P., Coffey, A., Delamont, S., Lofland, J., and Lofland, L. (Eds) (2007). *Handbook of Ethnography*. Sage.

Augurzky, B., Beivers, A., Breidenbach, P., Budde, R., Emde, A., Haering, A. et al (2018). *Notfallversorgung in Deutschland: Projektbericht im Auftrag der Kassenärztlichen Bundesvereinigung* (RWI Projektberichte, Issue).

Auyero, J. (2011). Patients of the State: An Ethnographic Account of Poor People's Waiting. *Latin American Research Review*, *46*(1), 5–29.

Back, L. (2015). Why Everyday Life Matters: Class, Community and Making Life Livable. *Sociology*, *49*(5), 820–36.

Baier, N., Geissler, A., Bech, M., Bernstein, D., Cowling, T.E., Jackson, T. et al (2019). Emergency and Urgent Care Systems in Australia, Denmark, England, France, Germany and the Netherlands – Analyzing Organization, Payment and Reforms. *Health Policy*, *123*(1), 1–10. https://doi.org/10.1016/j.healthpol.2018.11.001

Ballestero, A. (2014). What Is in a Percentage? Calculation as the Poetic Translation of Human Rights. *Indiana Journal of Global Legal Studies*, *21*(1), 27–53. https://doi.org/10.2979/indjglolegstu.21.1.27

Barman, E. (2013). Classificatory Struggles in the Nonprofit Sector: The Formation of the National Taxonomy of Exempt Entities, 1969–1987. *Social Science History*, *37*(1), 103–41. https://doi.org/10.1017/S0145553200010580

Barnard, A.V. (2019). Bureaucratically Split Personalities: (Re)Ordering the Mentally Disordered in the French State. *Theory and Society*, *48*(5), 753–84. https://doi.org/10.1007/s11186-019-09364-2

Barone, A.D., Yoels, W.C., and Clair, J.M. (1999). How Physicians View Caregivers: Simmel in the Examination Room. *Sociological Perspectives*, *42*(4), 673–90. https://doi.org/10.2307/1389579

Baumann, A., Sellin, S., and Breckwoldt, J. (2009). Standardisierte Notruf-Abfragesysteme für die Leitstelle. *Notfallmedizin up2date*, *4*(03), 261–77.

BBC (2018). Emergency Departments under 'Severe Pressure'. https://www.bbc.com/news/uk-northern-ireland-42552377

Behringer, W., Buergi, U., Christ, M., Dodt, C., and Hogan, B. (2013). Fünf Thesen zur Weiterentwicklung der Notfallmedizin in Deutschland, Österreich und der Schweiz. *Notfall + Rettungsmedizin*, *16*(8), 625–26. https://doi.org/10.1007/s10049-013-1821-8

Berchet, C. (2015). *Emergency Care Services: Trends, Drivers and Interventions to Manage the Demand.* OECD Health Working Papers, Issue.

Berger, E., Rödiger, H., and Busse, R. (2024). Reform der Notfallversorgung und des Rettungswesens. In J. Klauber, J. Wasem, A. Beivers, C. Mostert, and D. Scheller-Kreinsen (Eds), *Krankenhaus-Report 2024: Strukturreform* (pp 210–22). Springer.

Betz, M., and O'Connell, L. (2014). Changing Doctor–Patient Relationships and the Rise in Concern for Accountability. *Social Problems*, *31*(1), 84–95. https://doi.org/10.2307/800411

Biehl, J. (2012). Care and Disregard. In D. Fassin (Ed.), *A Companion to Moral Anthropology* (pp 242–63). Wiley-Blackwell.

Blokland, T. (2012). Blaming Neither the Undeserving Poor Nor the Revanchist Middle Classes: A Relational Approach to Marginalization. *Urban Geography*, *33*(4), 488–507.

Blokland, T. (2017). *Community as Urban Practice*. Polity Press.

Blokland, T. (2019). 'They Got a Project Mentality': Theorizing Neighborhood Dis-Identification and the Paradox of Belonging through the Lens of 'the Ghetto'. *Die Erde*, *150*(2), 101–12.

Blokland, T., Krüger, D., Vief, R., and Schultze, H. (2021). Where We Turn to: Rethinking Networks, Urban Space, and Research Methods. In A. Million, C. Haid, I. Castillo Ulloa, and N. Baur (Eds), *Spatial Transformations: Kaleidoscopic Perspectives on the Refiguration of Spaces* (pp 258–68). Routledge.

Blümel, M., Spranger, A., Achstetter, K., Maresso, A., and Busse, R. (2020). *Germany – Health System Review 2020* (Vol. 22). WHO Regional Office for Europe.

Boltanski, L., and Thévenot, L. (1999). The Sociology of Critical Capacity. *European Journal of Social Theory*, *2*(3), 359–77. https://doi.org/10.1177/136843199002003010

Booker, M.J., Shaw, A.R.G., and Purdy, S. (2015). Why Do Patients with 'Primary Care Sensitive' Problems Access Ambulance Services? A Systematic Mapping Review of the Literature. *BMJ Open*, *5*(5), 1–10. https://doi.org/10.1136/bmjopen-2015-007726

Bourdieu, P. (1977). *Outline of a Theory of Practice* (R. Nice, Trans.). Cambridge University Press. https://doi.org/10.1017/CBO9780511812507

Bourdieu, P. (1986). The Forms of Capital. In J.G. Richardson (Ed.), *Handbook of Theory and Research for the Sociology of Education* (pp 241–58). Greenwood Press.

Bourdieu, P. (1990). *The Logic of Practice*. Stanford University Press.

Bourdieu, P. (1994). Rethinking the State: Genesis and Structure of the Bureaucratic Field. *Sociological Theory*, *12*(1), 1–18. https://doi.org/10.2307/202032

Bourdieu, P. (2000). *Pascalian Meditations*. Polity Press.

Bourdieu, P. (2011). The Forms of Capital. In S.J. Ball (Ed.), *The RoutledgeFalmer Reader in Sociology of Education* (pp 15–29). Routledge.

Bourdieu, P. (2014). *On the State: Lectures at the College de France, 1989–1992*. Polity Press.

Bourdieu, P. (2018a). *Classification Struggles: General Sociology* (Vol. 1). Polity.

Bourdieu, P. (2018b). Social Space and the Genesis of Appropriated Physical Space. *International Journal of Urban and Regional Research*, *42*(1), 106–14. https://doi.org/10.1111/1468-2427.12534

Bourdieu, P., and Wacquant, L. (1992). *An Invitation to Reflexive Sociology*. Polity Press.

Bourgois, P., Holmes, S., Sue, K., and Quesada, J. (2017). Structural Vulnerability: Operationalizing the Concept to Address Health Disparities in Clinical Care. *Acad Med*, *92*(3), 299–307.

Brady, M. (2012). Pre-Hospital Psychosocial Care: Changing Attitudes. *Journal of Paramedic Practice*, *4*(9), 516–25. https://doi.org/10.12968/jpar.2012.4.9.516

Breuer, F., Brettschneider, P., Poloczek, S., Pommerenke, C., Wolff, J., and Dahmen, J. (2024). Quo vadis, gemeinsames Notfallleitsystem? *Notfall + Rettungsmedizin*, *27*(8), 640–49. https://doi.org/10.1007/s10049-022-01073-1

Breuer, F., Pommerenke, C., Wollenhaupt, L., Brettschneider, P., and Poloczek, S. (2020). Vorkommen von Frequent Usern und Frequent Callern in einem großstädtischen Rettungsdienst: Indikatoren eines unzureichenden Gesundheits- und Sozialsystems? *Notfall + Rettungsmedizin*, *23*(2), 122–31. https://doi.org/10.1007/s10049-019-0600-6

Brosnan, C. (2009). Pierre Bourdieu and the Theory of Medical Education: Thinking 'Relationally' about Medical Students and Medical Curricula. In C. Brosnan and B.S. Turner (Eds), *Handbook of the Sociology of Medical Education* (pp 51–68). Routledge. https://doi.org/http://ndl.ethernet.edu.et/bitstream/123456789/10191/1/110.pdf.pdf#page=66

Brown, A.D., Gabriel, Y., and Gherardi, S. (2009). Storytelling and Change: An Unfolding Story. *Organization*, *16*(3), 323–33. https://doi.org/10.1177/1350508409102298

Brown, P., Lyson, M., and Jenkins, T. (2011). From Diagnosis to Social Diagnosis. *Social Science & Medicine*, *73*(6), 939–43. https://doi.org/10.1016/j.socscimed.2011.05.031

Buchbinder, M. (2017). Keeping Out and Getting In: Reframing Emergency Department Gatekeeping as Structural Competence. *Sociology of Health & Illness*, *39*(7), 1166–79. https://doi.org/10.1111/1467-9566.12566

Bundesministerium für Gesundheit (BMG) (2023). Vierte Stellungnahme und Empfehlung der Regierungskommission für eine moderne und bedarfsgerechte. KrankenhausversorgungReform der Notfall- und Akut versorgung in Deutschland Integrierte Notfallzentren und Integrierte Leitstellen. https://www.bundesgesundheitsministerium.de/fileadmin/Dateien/3_Downloads/K/Krankenhausreform/Vierte_Stellungnahme_Regierungskommission_Notfall_ILS_und_INZ.pdf

Bundesministerium für Gesundheit (BMG) (2024a). Eckpunkte zur Reform der Notfallversorgung. https://www.bundesgesundheitsministerium.de/fileadmin/Dateien/3_Downloads/N/Notfallversorgung/Eckpunkte_Notfallreform_16.01.2024.pdf

Bundesministerium für Gesundheit (BMG) (2024b). Entwurf eines Gesetzes zur Reform der Notfallversorgung. https://www.bundesgesundheitsministerium.de/fileadmin/Dateien/3_Downloads/Gesetze_und_Verordnungen/GuV/N/GE_Notfallreform_Kabinett.pdf

Bundesministerium für Gesundheit (BMG) (2025). Referentenentwurf des Bundesministeriums für Gesundheit: Entwurf eines Gesetzes zur Reform der Notfallversorgung. https://www.bundesgesundheitsministerium.de/service/gesetze-und-verordnungen/detail/notfallreform

Bundesverbandes der Ärztlichen Leiter Rettungsdienst Deutschland (ÄRLD) e.V. (2015). *Umgang mit Alarmierungen des Rettungsdienstes zu banalen Erkrankungen und Verletzungen.* https://www.aelrd.de/index.php/downloads/category/23-transportverweigerung?download=17:20150421-stn-bv-aelrd-transportverweigerung

Bündnis Pro Rettungsdienst (2022). *Forderung einer Reform der Notfallversorgung*

Burawoy, M. (2019). Empiricism and Its Fallacies. *Contexts*, *18*(1), 47–53. https://doi.org/10.1177/1536504219830677

Busse, R., and Blümel, M. (2014). Germany – Health System Review: Health Systems in Transition. *WHO Regional Office for Europe*, *16*(2), 1–296.

Busse, R., Blümel, M., Knieps, F., and Bärnighausen, T. (2017). Statutory Health Insurance in Germany: A Health System Shaped by 135 Years of Solidarity, Self-Governance, and Competition. *The Lancet*, *390*(10097), 882–97. https://doi.org/10.1016/S0140-6736(17)31280-1

Calnan, M. (2015). Eliot Freidson: Sociological Narratives of Professionalism and Modern Medicine. In F. Collyer (Ed.), *The Palgrave Handbook of Social Theory in Health, Illness and Medicine* (pp 287–305). Palgrave Macmillan UK. https://doi.org/10.1057/9781137355621_19

Carret, M.L., Fassa, A.C., and Domingues, M.R. (2009). Inappropriate Use of Emergency Services: A Systematic Review of Prevalence and Associated Factors. *Cad Saude Publica*, *25*(1), 7–28. https://doi.org/10.1590/s0102-311x2009000100002

Carter, M. (2014). Vocation and Altruism in Nursing: The Habits of Practice. *Nursing Ethics*, *21*(6), 695–706. https://doi.org/10.1177/0969733013516159

Čartolovni, A., Stolt, M., Scott, P.A., and Suhonen, R. (2021). Moral Injury in Healthcare Professionals: A Scoping Review and Discussion. *Nursing Ethics*, *28*(5), 590–602. https://doi.org/10.1177/0969733020966776

Chappell, N.L., and Funk, L.M. (2011). Social Support, Caregiving, and Aging. *Canadian Journal on Aging / La Revue canadienne du vieillissement*, *30*(3), 355–70. https://doi.org/10.1017/S0714980811000316

Charmaz, K. (1999). Stories of Suffering: Subjective Tales and Research Narratives. *Qualitative Health Research*, *9*(3), 362–82. https://doi.org/10.1177/104973239900900306

Chinn, D. (2011). Critical Health Literacy: A Review and Critical Analysis. *Social Science & Medicine*, *73*(1), 60–7.

Christ, M., Grossmann, F., Winter, D., Bingisser, R., and Platz, E. (2010). Modern Triage in the Emergency Department. *Deutsches Ärzteblatt International*, *107*(50), 892–8.

Clayton, J., Donovan, C., and Merchant, J. (2015). Emotions of Austerity: Care and Commitment in Public Service Delivery in the North East of England. *Emotion, Space and Society*, *14*, 24–32. https://doi.org/10.1016/j.emospa.2014.11.004

Collyer, F.M. (2018). Envisaging the Healthcare Sector as a Field: Moving from Talcott Parsons to Pierre Bourdieu [journal article]. *Social Theory & Health*, *16*(2), 111–26. https://doi.org/10.1057/s41285-017-0046-1

Collyer, F.M., Willis, K.F., Franklin, M., Harley, K., and Short, S.D. (2015). Healthcare Choice: Bourdieu's Capital, Habitus and Field. *Current Sociology*, *63*(5), 685–99. https://doi.org/10.1177/0011392115590082

Coster, J.E., Turner, J.K., Bradbury, D., and Cantrell, A. (2017). Why Do People Choose Emergency and Urgent Care Services? A Rapid Review Utilizing a Systematic Literature Search and Narrative Synthesis. *Acad Emerg Med*, *24*(9), 1137–49. https://doi.org/10.1111/acem.13220

Dahmen, J., Brettschneider, P., Poloczek, S., Pommerenke, C., Wollenhaupt, L., and Breuer, F. (2021). 'Warum wird der Notruf 112 gewählt?' – Befragung zum Notrufverhalten der Berliner Bevölkerung. *Notfall + Rettungsmedizin*. https://doi.org/10.1007/s10049-021-00954-1

David-Barrett, T., Kertesz, J., Rotkirch, A., Ghosh, A., Bhattacharya, K., Monsivais, D. et al (2016). Communication with Family and Friends across the Life Course. *PLOS ONE*, *11*(11), e0165687. https://doi.org/10.1371/journal.pone.0165687

de Vaan, M., and Stuart, T. (2022). Gender in the Markets for Expertise. *American Sociological Review*, *87*(3), 443–77. https://doi.org/10.1177/00031224221087374

Dejean, D., Giacomini, M., Welsford, M., Schwartz, L., and Decicca, P. (2016). Inappropriate Ambulance Use: A Qualitative Study of Paramedics' Views [Utilisation inadéquate de l'ambulance: étude qualitative du point de vue des ambulanciers]. *Healthcare Policy*, *11*(3), 67–79.

Dejure (2022). *Ambulante Behandlung durch Krankenhäuser bei Unterversorgung*. https://dejure.org/gesetze/SGB_V/116a.html

Desmond, M. (2006). Becoming a Firefighter. *Ethnography*, 7(4), 387–421. https://doi.org/10.1177/1466138106073142

Desmond, M. (2007). *On The Fireline: Living and Dying with Wildland Firefighters*. University of Chicago Press.

Desmond, M. (2014). Relational Ethnography. *Theory and Society*, *43*(5), 547–79.

Deutsches Ärzteblatt. (2018). Notaufnahme: Gassen spricht sich für Gebühr aus. https://www.aerzteblatt.de/news/notaufnahme-gassen-spricht-sich-fuer-gebuehr-aus-a59f19ed-f5ca-4f8c-9e50-56b36c35ab79

Deutsches Ärzteblatt. (2023a). Gesundheitsexperten sehen schwere Mängel im Rettungswesen. https://www.aerzteblatt.de/search/result/ef531025-d005-4913-8278-869e4111c133?q=rettungsdienst+protest

Deutsches Ärzteblatt. (2023b). Streik legt britischen Rettungsdienst lahm. https://www.aerzteblatt.de/news/streik-legt-britischen-rettungsdienst-lahm-5ac53205-44a5-48f8-b487-f84f3628aa17

Deutsches Ärzteblatt. (2023c). Verdi ruft zu Warnstreiks im Gesundheitswesen auf. https://www.aerzteblatt.de/search/result/41e2dd1e-7994-4902-a2bd-981c6e758c8f?q=rettungsdienst+protest

Dhand, A., Luke, D., Lang, C., Tsiaklides, M., Feske, S., and Lee, J.-M. (2019). Social Networks and Risk of Delayed Hospital Arrival After Acute Stroke. *Nature Communications*, *10*(1), 1206. https://doi.org/10.1038/s41467-019-09073-5

DiCicco-Bloom, B., and Gibson, D.R. (2010). More than a Game: Sociological Theory from the Theories of Games. *Sociological Theory*, *28*(3), 247–271. https://doi.org/10.1111/j.1467-9558.2010.01377.x

Dodier, N., and Camus, A. (1998). Openness and Specialisation: Dealing with Patients in a Hospital Emergency Service. *Sociology of Health & Illness*, *20*(4), 413–44. https://doi.org/10.1111/1467-9566.00109

Dodson, L. (2009). *The Moral Underground: How Ordinary Americans Subvert an Unfair* Economy. The New Press.

Döring, A., and Paul, F. (2010). The German Healthcare System. *The EPMA journal*, *1*(4), 535–47. https://doi.org/10.1007/s13167-010-0060-z

Douglass, T., and Calnan, M. (2016). Trust Matters for Doctors? Towards an Agenda for Research. *Social Theory & Health*, *14*(4), 393–413. https://doi.org/10.1057/s41285-016-0010-5

Dressler, J.L. (2017). Gewalttätige Übergriffe auf Rettungskräfte. *forum kriminalprävention*, *3*, 3–6.

Dück, J. (2022). *Soziale Reproduktion in der Krise: Sorgekämpfe in Krankenhäusern und Kitas*. Beltz Juventa.

Duneier, M. (2002). What Kind of Combat Sport Is Sociology? *American Journal of Sociology*, *107*(6), 1551–76. https://doi.org/10.1086/342925

Dykstra, P.A. (2015). Aging and Social Support. In G. Ritzer (Ed.), *The Blackwell Encyclopedia of Sociology*. https://doi.org/10.1002/9781405165518.wbeosa033.pub2

Ellebrecht, N. (2009). Triage: Charakteristika und Gegenwart eines Ordnungsstiftenden Verfahrens. *Sociologia Internationalis*, *47*(2), 229–57. https://doi.org/10.3790/sint.47.2.229

Ellebrecht, N. (2020). *Organisierte Rettung Studien zur Soziologie des Notfalls*. Springer.

Emirbayer, M. (1997). Manifesto for a Relational Sociology. *American Journal of Sociology*, *103*(2), 281–317.

Emirbayer, M., and Johnson, V. (2008). Bourdieu and Organizational Analysis [journal article]. *Theory and Society*, *37*(1), 1–44. https://doi.org/10.1007/s11186-007-9052-y

Faculty of Humanities and Social Sciences (2018). *Regulations for the Ethics Committee of the Faculty of Humanities and Social Sciences*. https://fakultaeten.hu-berlin.de/de/ksb/die-fakultaet/rat_kommissionen/ethikkommission/1_16_2018__ethiksatzung_ksbf_druck_englisch.pdf

Fahimi, J., and Goldfrank, L. (2019). Principles of Social Emergency Medicine. *Annals of Emergency Medicine*, *74*(5), S6–S10. https://doi.org/10.1016/j.annemergmed.2019.08.432

Fainzang, S. (2002). Lying, Secrecy and Power within the Doctor-Patient Relationship. *Anthropology & Medicine*, *9*(2), 117–33. https://doi.org/10.1080/1364847022000034574

Fassin, D. (2008). The Elementary Forms of Care: An Empirical Approach to Ethics in a South African Hospital. *Social Science & Medicine*, *67*(2), 262–70. https://doi.org/10.1016/j.socscimed.2008.03.044

Fassin, D. (2018). *Life: A Critical User's Manual*. Polity Press.

Federal Committee (2022). *Patient involvement*. https://www.g-ba.de/english/structure/patient/

Fine, G.A., Montemurro, B., Semora, B., Stalp, M.C., Claussen, D.S., and Sierra, Z. (1998). Social Order through a Prism: Color as Collective Representation. *Sociological Inquiry*, *68*(4), 443–57. https://doi.org/10.1111/j.1475-682X.1998.tb00479.x

Fink, M. (2021). *Forget Burial: HIV Kinship, Disability, and Queer/Trans Narratives of Care*. Rutgers University Press.

Fleischmann, T., and Amler, N. (2014). Ökonomie und Psychologie des Wartens. *Deutsches Ärzteblatt*, *111*(39), 1642–44.

Frankfurter Allgemeine Zeitung (2018). Überfüllte Kliniken: Notaufnahmen am Limit. *Frankfurter Allgemeine Zeitung*. https://www.faz.net/aktuell/rhein-main/kliniken-leiden-unter-ueberfuellung-15663266.html

Freidson, E. (2001). *Professionalism, the Third Logic*. The University of Chicago Press.

Friedman, A., and Pauly, M. (2020). Why the Emergency Room Is Always Crowded And What We Can Do about It. *The Philadelphia Inquirer*. https://www.inquirer.com/health/expert-opinions/emergency-room-overcrowded-solutions-20200106.html

Gerlinger, T. (2017). *Strukturen und Versorgungsformen*. bpb. https://www.bpb.de/themen/gesundheit/gesundheitspolitik/251980/strukturen-und-versorgungsformen/

Gerlinger, T. (2021). Krankenhäuser in Deutschland: Strukturen – Probleme – Reformen. *APUZ, 30-21*(71), 9–16.

Gerst, T. (2015). 60 Jahre Kassenärztliche Bundesvereinigung: Der lange Weg zum Kassenarztrecht. *Deutsches Ärzteblatt, 10*(October 2015), 445–446.

González de la Rocha, M. (2020). Of Morals and Markets: Social Exchange and Poverty in Contemporary Urban Mexico. *The ANNALS of the American Academy of Political and Social Science, 689*(1), 26–45. https://doi.org/10.1177/0002716220916700

Gordon, J.A. (1999). The Hospital Emergency Department as a Social Welfare Institution. *Annals of Emergency Medicine, 33*(3), 321–25. https://doi.org/10.1016/S0196-0644(99)70369-0

Gordon, J.A. (2001). Cost-Benefit Analysis of Social Work Services in the Emergency Department: A Conceptual Model. *Academic Emergency Medicine, 8*(1), 54–60. https://doi.org/10.1111/j.1553-2712.2001.tb00552.x

Gräff, I., Goldschmidt, B., Glien, P., Bogdanow, M., Fimmers, R., Hoeft, A. et al (2014). The German Version of the Manchester Triage System and its Quality Criteria: First Assessment of Validity and Reliability. *PLOS ONE, 9*(2), e88995. https://doi.org/10.1371/journal.pone.0088995

Gritti, F. (2018). Überlastete Feuerwehren: 'Letztlich leidet der Bürger'. *Spiegel.* https://www.spiegel.de/panorama/gesellschaft/rettungsdienst-zahl-der-einsaetze-steigt-von-jahr-zu-jahr-a-1203793.html

Günther, A., Schmid, S., Bruns, A., Kleinschmidt, T., Bartkiewicz, T., and Harding, U. (2017). Ambulante Kontakte mit dem Rettungsdienst [journal article]. *Notfall + Rettungsmedizin, 20*(6), 477–85. https://doi.org/10.1007/s10049-017-0268-8

Hage, G. (2011). Social Gravity: Pierre Bourdieu's Phenomenological Social Physics. In G. Hage and E. Kowal (Eds), *Force Movement, Intensity: The Newtonian Imagination in the Social Sciences* (pp 80–92). Melbourne University Press.

Hammersley, M. (2018). Book Review: Steven Lubet, Interrogating Ethnography: Why Evidence Matters. *Qualitative Research, 0*(0), 1468794118808202. https://doi.org/10.1177/1468794118808202

Hammersley, M., and Atkinson, P. (2010). *Ethnography: Principles in Practice.* Routledge.

Hanke, S. (2021). *Der Ärztestellen-Jahresrückblick: Der Arbeitsmarkt für Mediziner im Jahr 2020.* https://aerztestellen.aerzteblatt.de/de/redaktion/jobwechsel-und-gehalt/aerztestellen-jahresrueckblick-2020

Hansen, H., Bourgois, P., and Drucker, E. (2014). Pathologizing Poverty: New Forms of Diagnosis, Disability, and Structural Stigma under Welfare Reform. *Soc Sci Med, 103*(February), 76–83.

Harrits, G.S., and Møller, M.Ø. (2011). Categories and Categorization: Towards a Comprehensive Sociological Framework. *Distinktion: Scandinavian Journal of Social Theory, 12*(2), 229–47.

Heimer, C.A., Coleman Petty, J., and Culyba, R.J. (2005). Risk and Rules: The 'Legalization' of Medicine. In B. Hutter and M. Power (Eds), *Organizational Encounters with Risk* (pp 92–131). Cambridge University Press.

Henckes, N., and Nurok, M. (2015). 'The First Pulse You Take is Your Own' – but Don't Forget Your Colleagues': Emotion Teamwork in Pre-Hospital Emergency Medical Services. *Sociology of Health & Illness*, *37*(7), 1023–38. https://doi.org/10.1111/1467-9566.12261

Hering, T., and Beerlage, I. (2004). Arbeitsbedingungen, Belastungen und Burnout im Rettungsdienst. *Notfall & Rettungsmedizin*, 7(6), 415–24. https://doi.org/10.1007/s10049-004-0681-7

Higashi, R.T., Tillack, A., Steinman, M.A., Johnston, C.B., and Harper, G.M. (2013). The 'Worthy' Patient: Rethinking the 'Hidden Curriculum' in Medical Education. *Anthropology & Medicine*, *20*(1), 13–23. https://doi.org/10.1080/13648470.2012.747595

Hillman, A. (2014). 'Why Must I Wait?' The Performance of Legitimacy in a Hospital Emergency Department. *Sociology of Health & Illness*, *36*(4), 485–99. https://doi.org/10.1111/1467-9566.12072

Hillman, A. (2016). Institutions of Care, Moral Proximity and Demoralisation: The Case of the Emergency Department. *Social Theory & Health*, *14*(1), 66–87. https://doi.org/10.1057/sth.2015.10

Holmes, S.M. (2007). Oaxacans Like to Work Bent Over: The Naturalization of Social Suffering among Berry Farm Workers. *International Migration*, *45*(3), 39–68. https://doi.org/10.1111/j.1468-2435.2007.00410.x

Holmes, S.M. (2013). *Fresh Fruit, Broken Bodies: Migrant Farmworkers in the United States*. University of California Press.

Holmes, S.M., and Ponte, M. (2011). En-case-ing the Patient: Disciplining Uncertainty in Medical Student Patient Presentations [journal article]. *Culture, Medicine, and Psychiatry*, *35*(2), 163–82. https://doi.org/10.1007/s11013-011-9213-3

Hölter, K. (2018). Feuerwehr-Protest in Berlin: 'Es bleibt nicht mal Zeit zum Essen'. https://www.spiegel.de/panorama/feuerwehr-protest-in-berlin-helfer-berichten-ueber-katastrophale-arbeitsbedingungen-a-00000000-0003-0001-0000-000002227674

Hoot, N.R., and Aronsky, D. (2008). Systematic Review of Emergency Department Crowding: Causes, Effects, and Solutions. *Annals of Emergency Medicine*, *52*(2), 126–136.e121. https://doi.org/10.1016/j.annemergmed.2008.03.014

Hudgins, A., and Rising, K.L. (2016). Fear, Vulnerability and Sacrifice: Drivers of Emergency Department Use and Implications for Policy. *Social Science & Medicine*, *169*, 50–7. https://doi.org/10.1016/j.socscimed.2016.09.030

Hupe, P. (2012). Autonomy in Health Care Practice: A Paradise Lost? In H. Dickinson and R. Mannion (Eds), *The Reform of Health Care: Shaping, Adapting and Resisting Policy Developments* (pp 37–50). Palgrave Macmillan UK. https://doi.org/10.1057/9780230355026_4

Hupe, P., and Hill, M. (2007). Street-Level Bureaucracy and Public Accountability. *Public Administration, 85*(2), 279–99. https://doi.org/10.1111/j.1467-9299.2007.00650.x

Huschke, S. (2014). Performing Deservingness: Humanitarian Health Care Provision for Migrants in Germany. *Social Science & Medicine, 120*, 352–9. https://doi.org/10.1016/j.socscimed.2014.04.046

Institute of Medicine Committee on Data Standards for Patient Safety (2004). In P. Aspden, J.M. Corrigan, J. Wolcott, and S.M. Erickson (Eds), *Patient Safety: Achieving a New Standard for Care*. National Academies Press (US) Copyright 2004 by the National Academy of Sciences. All rights reserved. https://doi.org/10.17226/10863

Jacobs, G., van Witteloostuijn, A., and Christe-Zeyse, J. (2013). A Theoretical Framework of Organizational Change. *Journal of Organizational Change Management, 26*(5), 772–92. https://doi.org/10.1108/JOCM-09-2012-0137

Jacobsson, K., Wallinder, Y., and Seing, I. (2020). Street-Level Bureaucrats Under New Managerialism: A Comparative Study of Agency Cultures and Caseworker Role Identities in Two Welfare State Bureaucracies. *Journal of Professions and Organization*, 7(3), 316–33. https://doi.org/10.1093/jpo/joaa015

Jeffery, R. (1979). Normal Rubbish: Deviant Patients in Casualty Departments. *Sociology of Health & Illness, 1*(1), 90–107. https://doi.org/10.1111/1467-9566.ep11006793

Jenkins, R. (2000). Categorization: Identity, Social Process and Epistemology. *Current Sociology, 48*(3), 7–25. https://doi.org/10.1177/0011392100048003003

Jensen, C., and Petersen, M.B. (2017). The Deservingness Heuristic and the Politics of Health Care. *American Journal of Political Science, 61*(1), 68–83. https://doi.org/10.1111/ajps.12251

Johannessen, L.E.F. (2017). Beyond Guidelines: Discretionary Practice in Face-to-Face Triage Nursing. *Sociology of Health & Illness, 39*(7), 1180–94. https://doi.org/10.1111/1467-9566.12578

Johannessen, L.E.F. (2018a). Narratives and Gatekeeping: Making Sense of Triage Nurses' Practice. *Sociology of Health & Illness, 40*(5), 892–906. https://doi.org/10.1111/1467-9566.12732

Johannessen, L.E.F. (2018b). Workplace Assimilation and Professional Jurisdiction: How Nurses Learn to Blur the Nursing-Medical Boundary. *Social Science & Medicine, 201*, 51–8. https://doi.org/10.1016/j.socscimed.2018.02.004

Johannessen, L.E.F. (2019a). The Commensuration of Pain: How Nurses Transform Subjective Experience Into Objective Numbers. *Social Science & Medicine, 233*, 38–46. https://doi.org/10.1016/j.socscimed.2019.05.042

Johannessen, L.E.F. (2019b). Negotiated Discretion: Redressing the Neglect of Negotiation in "Street-Level Bureaucracy". *Symbolic Interaction, 42*(4), 513–38. https://doi.org/10.1002/symb.451

Johnson, K.D., and Winkelman, C. (2011). The Effect of Emergency Department Crowding on Patient Outcomes: A Literature Review. *Advanced Emergency Nursing Journal, 33*(1), 39–54.

Joseph, A.E., and Hallman, B.C. (1998). Over the Hill and Far Away: Distance as a Barrier to the Provision of Assistance to Elderly Relatives. *Social Science & Medicine, 46*(6), 631–9. https://doi.org/10.1016/S0277-9536(97)00181-0

Jutel, A., and Nettleton, S. (2011). Towards a Sociology of Diagnosis: Reflections and Opportunities. *Social Science & Medicine, 73*(6), 793–800. https://doi.org/10.1016/j.socscimed.2011.07.014

Kalitzkus, V., Wilm, S., and Matthiessen, P.F. (2009). Narrative Medizin: Was ist es, Was bringt es, Wie setzt man es um? *Zeitschrift für Allgemeinmedizin, 85*(2), 60–6.

Karutz, H. (2014). Der psychosoziale Notfall: Für den Rettungsdienst ein Fehleinsatz? *Rettungsdienst, 37*(7), 32–7.

Karutz, H., Overhagen, M., and Stum, J. (2013). Psychische Belastungen im Wachalltag von Rettungsdienstmitarbeitern und Feuerwehrleuten. *Prävention und Gesundheitsförderung, 8*(3), 204–11. https://doi.org/10.1007/s11553-012-0373-y

Kassenärztliche Vereinigung Berlin (2017). Diskussion zu Notfallversorgung nimmt Fahrt auf: Einigkeit über Reformbedarf. *KV Blatt, 12.2017*.

Kawakami, C., Ohshige, K., Kubota, K., and Tochikubo, O. (2007). Influence of Socioeconomic Factors on Medically Unnecessary Ambulance Calls. *BMC Health Services Research*, 7(1), 120. https://doi.org/10.1186/1472-6963-7-120

Knorr Cetina, K. (2009). Jenseits der Aufklärung. Die Entstehung der Kultur des Lebens. In M.G. Weiß (Ed.), *Bios und Zoë. Die menschliche Natur im Zeitalter ihrer technischen Reproduzierbarkeit* (pp 55–71). Suhrkamp.

Koch, I. (2020). The Guardians of the Welfare State: Universal Credit, Welfare Control and the Moral Economy of Frontline Work in Austerity Britain. *Sociology, 0*(0), 0038038520936981. https://doi.org/10.1177/0038038520936981

Koch, M., Piñeiro, E., and Pasche, N. (2019). 'We Are a Service, Not an Authority': Multiple Institutional Logics in a Swiss Youth Welfare Office. An Ethnographic Case Study From Street-Level Bureaucracy [child welfare; social work; street-level bureaucracy; ethnography; new institutionalism; multiple institutional logics; Switzerland]. *Forum Qualitative Social Research, 20*(2). https://doi.org/10.17169/fqs-20.2.3045

Kraaijvanger, N., van Leeuwen, H., Rijpsma, D., and Edwards, M. (2016). Motives for self-referral to the emergency department: a systematic review of the literature. *BMC Health Serv Res, 16*(1), 685. https://doi.org/10.1186/s12913-016-1935-z

Kristensen, S.M., Ersbøll, K.A., Ahlmark, N., and Thomsen, T.T. (2018). The Sociolance: A Mobile Clinic Requested Through Emergency Medical Dispatch Center Serving Socially Vulnerable and Homeless People in the Capital City of Denmark. *Revue d'Épidémiologie et de Santé Publique, 66*, S371. https://doi.org/10.1016/j.respe.2018.05.363

Krüger, D. (2023). *'It Has Become Normal to Call 112': Classificatory Struggles over the Increased Use of Emergency Care in Urgencity.* Humboldt-Universität zu Berlin.

Krüger, D. (2024). Homeless Clients' Circulation in Emergency Care: Rethinking Poverty Governance as Urban Impasse. *Tijdschrift voor Economische en Sociale Geografie, 115*(2), 221–33. https://doi.org/10.1111/tesg.12601

Krüger, D., and Schuster, A. (Eds). (2025). *Coordinated Care.* Intercomverlag.

Krüger, D., Voss, M., and Seidelsohn, K. (2017). Fragmentierte Sicherheit: Zur Produktion und Reproduktion von (Un-)Sicherheitsräumen in Städten [journal article]. *Soziale Probleme, 28*(2), 285–99. https://doi.org/10.1007/s41059-017-0037-4

Kühl, S., Strodtholz, P., and Taffertshofer, A. (Eds) (2009). *Handbuch Methoden der Organisationsforschung: Quantitative und Qualitative Methoden.* VS Verlag für Sozialwissenschaften.

Kuhlmann, E., Allsop, J., and Saks, M. (2009). Professional Governance and Public Control: A Comparison of Healthcare in the United Kingdom and Germany. *Current Sociology, 57*(4), 511–28. https://doi.org/10.1177/0011392109104352

Lach, H.W. (2005). Incidence and Risk Factors for Developing Fear of Falling in Older Adults. *Public Health Nursing, 22*(1), 45–52. https://doi.org/10.1111/j.0737-1209.2005.22107.x

Lamont, M. (1992). *Money, Morals, and Manners: The Culture of the French and American Upper-Middle Class.* University of Chicago Press.

Lamont, M. (2012). How Has Bourdieu Been Good to Think With? The Case of the United States. *Sociological Forum, 27*(1), 228–37. https://doi.org/10.1111/j.1573-7861.2011.01309.x

Lamont, M., and Molnár, V. (2002). The Study of Boundaries in the Social Sciences. *Annual Review of Sociology*, *28*, 167–95.

Lara-Millán, A. (2014). Public Emergency Room Overcrowding in the Era of Mass Imprisonment. *American Sociological Review*, *79*(5), 866–87. https://doi.org/10.1177/0003122414549552

Lara-Millán, A. (2017). States as a Series of People Exchanges. In A.S. Orloff and K.J. Morgan (Eds), *The Many Hands of the State: Theorizing Political Authority and Social Control* (pp 81–102). Cambridge University Press. https://doi.org/10.1017/9781316471586.004

Lara-Millán, A. (2021). *Redistributing the Poor: Jails, Hospitals, and the Crisis of Law and Fiscal Austerity*. Oxford University Press.

Leber, W.-D., and Wasem, J. (2016). Ambulante Krankenhausleistungen: Ein Überblick, eine Trendanalyse und einige ordnungspolitische Anmerkungen. In J. Klauber, M. Geraedts, J. Friedrich, and J. Wasem (Eds), *Krankenhaus-Report 2016: Ambulant im Krankenhaus* (pp 3–28). Wissenschaftliches Institut der AOK (WIdO).

Legg, D., A. Fischer-Rosinsky, F. Holzinger, M. Möckel and A. Slagman (2022). Overcoming Terminological Inconsistency in the Study of Emergency Department Attendees Who Do Not Require Clinically Defined Emergency care. *European Journal of Emergency Medicine*, *29*(6).

Leong, E. (2013). Collecting Knowledge for the Family: Recipes, Gender and Practical Knowledge in the Early Modern English Household. *Centaurus*, *55*(2), 81–103. https://doi.org/10.1111/1600-0498.12019

Leong, E. (2018). *Recipes and Everyday Knowledge: Medicine, Science, and the Household in Early Modern England*. University of Chicago Press.

Lindner, G., and Woitok, B.K. (2021). Emergency Department Overcrowding. *Wiener Klinische Wochenschrift*, *133*(5), 229–33. https://doi.org/10.1007/s00508-019-01596-7

Lindner, T. (2022). *Gewalt gegen in Notaufnahmen beschäftigtes Personal*. Charité-Universitätsmedizin Berlin.

Lipsky, M. (1980). *Street-Level Bureaucracy: Dilemmas of the Individual in Public Services*. Russell Sage.

Lipsky, M. (2010). *Street-Level Bureaucracy: Dilemmas of the Individual in Public Services*. Russell Sage.

Lockett, A., Currie, G., Finn, R., Martin, G., and Waring, J. (2014). The Influence of Social Position on Sensemaking about Organizational Change. *Academy of Management Journal*, *57*(4), 1102–29. https://doi.org/10.5465/amj.2011.0055

Lofland, J., and Lofland, L.H. (1995). *Analyzing Social Settings: A Guide to Qualitative Observation and Analysis*. Wadsworth.

Lopes, S., Soares, P., Santos Sousa, J., Rocha, J.V., Boto, P., and Santana, R. (2023). Effect of the COVID-19 Pandemic on the Frequency of Emergency Department Visits in Portugal: An Interrupted Time Series Analysis until July 2021. *JACEP Open*, *4*(1), e12864. https://doi.org/10.1002/emp2.12864

Lorenzen, J.-M., and Zifonun, D. (2012). Das Eigengewicht der Institutionen und die Zentralität der Laien: Anmerkungen zur Feldtheorie Pierre Bourdieus *SWS-Rundschau*, *52*(1), 92–108.

Loveman, M. (2005). The Modern State and the Primitive Accumulation of Symbolic Power. *American Journal of Sociology*, *110*(6), 1651–83. https://doi.org/10.1086/428688

Lowthian, J.A., Cameron, P.A., Stoelwinder, J.U., Curtis, A., Currell, A., Cooke, M.W., and McNeil, J.J. (2011). Increasing Utilisation of Emergency Ambulances. *Australian Health Review*, *35*(1), 63–9. https://doi.org/10.1071/AH09866

Lowthian, J.A., Curtis, A.J., Cameron, P.A., Stoelwinder, J.U., Cooke, M.W., and McNeil, J.J. (2011). Systematic Review of Trends in Emergency Department Attendances: An Australian Perspective. *Emergency Medicine Journal*, *28*(5), 373. https://doi.org/10.1136/emj.2010.099226

Lubet, S. (2018). *Interrogating Ethnography: Why Evidence Matters*. Oxford University Press.

Luhmann, N. (1979). *Trust and Power: Two Works by Niklas Luhmann, intr. G. Poggi*. John Wiley and Sons. (Orig. pub. 1968)

Luiz, T. (2008). Der psychosoziale Notfall [journal article]. *Notfall + Rettungsmedizin*, *11*(8), 547–51. https://doi.org/10.1007/s10049-008-1106-9

Luiz, T., Schmitt, T.K., and Madler, C. (2002). Der Notarzt als Manager sozialer Krisen. *Notfall + Rettungsmedizin*, *5*(7), 505–11. https://doi.org/10.1007/s10049-002-0502-9

Lupton, D. (2013). The Digitally Engaged Patient: Self-Monitoring and Self-Care in the Digital Health Era. *Social Theory & Health*, *11*(3), 256–70. https://doi.org/10.1057/sth.2013.10

Lupton, D., and Jutel, A. (2015). 'It's Like Having a Physician in Your Pocket!' A Critical Analysis of Self-Diagnosis Smartphone Apps. *Social Science & Medicine*, *133*, 128–35. https://doi.org/10.1016/j.socscimed.2015.04.004

Luzio, G.D. (2004). The Irresistible Decline of the Medical Profession? An Empirical Investigation of Its Autonomy and Economic Situation in the Changing German Welfare State. *German Politics*, *13*(3), 419–48. https://doi.org/10.1080/0964400042000287446

Luzio, G.D. (2006). A Sociological Concept of Client Trust. *Current Sociology*, *54*(4), 549–64. https://doi.org/10.1177/0011392106065087

Mangiapane, S., Czihal, T., and von St–illfried, D. (2021). Entwicklung der ambulanten Notfallversorgung in Deutschland von 2009 bis 2020. *Zi-Paper*, *16/2021*.

Margies, N. (2021). *Emotions and Social Change: Feeling Hysteresis in Post-Crisis Spain*. Humboldt-Universität zu Berlin.

Margies, N. (2024). *Emotions in Crisis: Youth and Social Change in Spain*. Policy Press.

Mattes, D., and Dinkelaker, S. (2019). Failing and Attuning in the Field: Introduction. In T. Stodulka, S. Dinkelaker, and F. Thajib (Eds), *Affective Dimensions of Fieldwork and Ethnography* (pp 227–231). Springer International Publishing. https://doi.org/10.1007/978-3-030-20831-8_20

Maynard-Moody, S., and Musheno, M. (2003). *Cops, Teachers, Counselors: Stories From The Front Lines of Public Service*. University of Michigan Press.

Maynard-Moody, S., and Portillo, S. (2011). Street-Level Bureaucracy Theory. In R.F. Durant (Ed.), *The Oxford Handbook of American Bureaucracy* (pp 1–28). Oxford University Press. https://doi.org/10.1093/oxfordhb/9780199238958.003.0011

Mayr, B. (2020). Structured or Protocol-Based Dispatching Programs [Strukturierte bzw. standardisierte Notrufabfrage: Leisten die Systeme tatsächlich, was sie vorgeben zu leisten?]. *Notfall & Rettungsmedizin*, 1–8. https://doi.org/10.1007/s10049-020-00733-4

McDonough, P. (2006). Habitus and the Practice of Public Service. *Work, Employment & Society*, *20*(4), 629–47.

McDonough, P., and Polzer, J. (2012). Habitus, Hysteresis, and Organizational Change in the Public Sector. *The Canadian Journal of Sociology*, *37*(4), 357–79.

McQuarrie, M., and Marwell, N.P. (2009). The Missing Organizational Dimension in Urban Sociology. *City & Community*, *8*(3), 247–68. https://doi.org/10.1111/j.1540-6040.2009.01288.x

MDR (2023). New Approaches in Emergency Services: Rescue for the Rescue Service? The Pilot Project 'Community Paramedic' Shows Initial Effects. https://www.mdr.de/nachrichten/sachsen-anhalt/dessau/wittenberg/pilotprojekt-rettungsdienst-gemeindenotfallsanitaeter-100.html

Merriam-Webster (n.d.). *Paramedical*. https://www.merriam-webster.com/dictionary/paramedical

Merton, R.K. (1976). *Sociological Ambivalence and Other Essays*. Free Press.

Metzl, J.M., and Hansen, H. (2014). Structural Competency: Theorizing a New Medical Engagement with Stigma and Inequality. *Social Science & Medicine*, *103*, 126–33. https://doi.org/10.1016/j.socscimed.2013.06.032

Mishler, E.G. (1984). *The Discourse of Medicine: dialectics of Medical Interviews*. Ablex Publishing.

Misztal, B. (1996). *Trust in Modern Societies: The Search for the Bases of Social Order*. Polity Press.

Misztal, B. (2001). Normality and Trust in Goffman's Theory of Interaction Order. *Sociological Theory*, *19*(3), 312–24. doi: 10.1111/0735-2751.00143

Misztal, B.A. (2005). The New Importance of the Relationship Between Formality and Informality. *Feminist Theory*, *6*(2), 173–94. https://doi.org/10.1177/1464700105053693

Misztal, B.A. (2015). *Multiple Normalities: Making Sense of Ways of Living*. Palgrave Macmillan.

Montgomery, B.J. (1980). A Capsule History of Us Emergency Medical Care. *JAMA*, *243*(10), 1019–21. https://doi.org/10.1001/jama.1980.03300360005002

Morley, C., Unwin, M., Peterson, G.M., Stankovich, J., and Kinsman, L. (2018). Emergency Department Crowding: A Systematic Review of Causes, Consequences and Solutions. *PLOS ONE*, *13*(8), 1–42. https://doi.org/10.1371/journal.pone.0203316

Moskop, J.C., Sklar, D.P., Geiderman, J.M., Schears, R.M., and Bookman, K.J. (2009). Emergency Department Crowding, Part 1: Concept, Causes, and Moral Consequences. *Ann Emerg Med*, *53*(5), 605–11. https://doi.org/10.1016/j.annemergmed.2008.09.019

Murphy, A.W. (1998). 'Inappropriate' Attenders at Accident and Emergency Departments I: Definition, Incidence and Reasons for Attendance. *Fam Pract*, *15*(1), 23–32. https://doi.org/10.1093/fampra/15.1.23

Nettleton, S. (2006). I Just Want Permission to Be Ill: Towards a Sociology of Medically Unexplained Symptoms. *Social Science & Medicine*, *62*(5), 1167–78.

Nettleton, S., and Burrows, R. (2003). E-Scaped Medicine? Information, Reflexivity and Health. *Critical Social Policy*, *23*(2), 165–85. https://doi.org/10.1177/0261018303023002003

Nettleton, S., Burrows, R., and Watt, I. (2008). Regulating Medical Bodies? The Consequences of the 'Modernisation' of the NHS and the Disembodiment of Clinical Knowledge. *Sociology of Health & Illness*, *30*(3), 333–48. https://doi.org/10.1111/j.1467-9566.2007.01057.x

Nettleton, S., Neale, J., and Pickering, L. (2013). 'I Just Want to Be Normal': An Analysis of Discourses of Normality Among Recovering Heroin Users. *Health*, *17*(2), 174–90. https://doi.org/10.1177/1363459312451182

Neubauer, G., Minartz, C., and Niedermeier, C. (2016). *Kritische Analyse des 'Gutachtens zur ambulanten Notfallversorgung im Krankenhaus: Fallkostenkalkulation und Strukturanalyse' der MCK in Kooperation mit der DGINA vom 17.02.2015. Expertise für das Zentralinstitut für die kassenärztliche Versorgung (Zi)*. https://www.zi.de/fileadmin/images/content/PDFs_alle/Expertise_Notfallversorgung_Endfassung.pdf

New Zealand Herald (2018). Emergency Departments Overwhelmed by Patients, not Meeting Targets. https://www.nzherald.co.nz/nz/emergency-departments-overwhelmed-by-patients-not-meeting-targets/RWHC4EG57EMKWFLZOKMCMZS6XY/

Newman, K. (2002). No Shame: The View from the Left Bank. *American Journal of Sociology, 107*(6), 1577–99. https://doi.org/10.1086/342993

Noordegraaf, M. (2007). From 'Pure' to 'Hybrid' Professionalism: Present-Day Professionalism in Ambiguous Public Domains. *Administration & Society, 39*(6), 761–85. https://doi.org/10.1177/0095399707304434

Nurok, M., and Henckes, N. (2009). Between Professional Values and the Social Valuation of Patients: The Fluctuating Economy of Pre-Hospital Emergency Work. *Social Science & Medicine, 68*(3), 504–10. https://doi.org/10.1016/j.socscimed.2008.11.001

Oslislo, S., Heintze, C., Schmiedhofer, M., Möckel, M., Schenk, L., and Holzinger, F. (2019). How to Decide Adequately? Qualitative Study of GPs' View on Decision-Making in Self-Referred and Physician-Referred Emergency Department Consultations in Berlin, Germany. *BMJ Open, 9*(4), e026786. https://doi.org/10.1136/bmjopen-2018-026786

Paling, S., Lambert, J., Clouting, J., González-Esquerré, J., and Auterson, T. (2020). Waiting Times in Emergency Departments: Exploring the Factors Associated with Longer Patient Waits for Emergency Care in England Using Routinely Collected Daily Data. *Emergency Medicine Journal, 37*(12), 781. https://doi.org/10.1136/emermed-2019-208849

Palmer, C.E. (1983). 'Trauma Junkies' and Street Work. *Urban Life, 12*(2), 162–83. https://doi.org/10.1177/0098303983012002003

Parsons, T. (1991 [1951]). *The Social System*. Routledge.

Peck, B.M., and Conner, S. (2011). Talking with Me or Talking at Me? The Impact of Status Characteristics on Doctor-Patient Interaction. *Sociological Perspectives, 54*(4), 547–67. https://doi.org/10.1525/sop.2011.54.4.547

Pescosolido, B.A. (1992). Beyond Rational Choice: The Social Dynamics of How People Seek Help. *American Journal of Sociology, 97*(4), 1096–138. https://doi.org/10.1086/229863

Przyborski, A., and Wohlrab-Sahr, M. (2009). *Qualitative Sozialforschung: Ein Arbeitsbuch*. De Gruyter.

Redelsteiner, C. (2018). Der Rettungsdienst als Gatekeeper medizinischer und sozialer Dienste. In A. Neumayr, M. Baubin, and A. Schinnerl (Eds), *Herausforderung Notfallmedizin: Innovation – Vision – Zukunft* (pp 107–17). Springer Berlin Heidelberg. https://doi.org/10.1007/978-3-662-56627-5_10

Rehbein, B., and Saalmann, G. (2014). Kapital (Capital). In G. Fröhlich and B. Rehbein (Eds), *Bourdieu-Handbuch: Leben – Werk – Wirkung* (pp 134–40). J.B. Metzler. https://doi.org/10.1007/978-3-476-01379-8_29

Reibling, N., and Wendt, C. (2012). Gatekeeping and Provider Choice in OECD Healthcare Systems. *Current Sociology, 60*(4), 489–505. https://doi.org/10.1177/0011392112438333

Rettet den Rettungsdienst (2022). *Unsere Forderungen an die Politik | Rettet den Rettungsdienst*

Rhodes, L.A. (1995). *Emptying Beds: The Work of an Emergency Psychiatric Unit*. University of California Press.

Rieder, C. (2025). Social Work in Emergency Departments – auch für Deutschland. *FORUM sozialarbeit + gesundheit, 2025*(2), 10–13.

Riedlinger, I., Fischer, G., Lämmel, N., and Höß, T. (2020). Leasing ist wie ein stummer Streik: Zeitarbeit in der Pflege. *AIS-Studien, 13*(2), 142–57. https://doi.org/10.21241/ssoar.70996

Riessen, R., Gries, A., Seekamp, A., Dodt, C., Kumle, B., and Busch, H.-J. (2015). Positionspapier für eine Reform der medizinischen Notfallversorgung in deutschen Notaufnahmen. *Notfall + Rettungsmedizin, 18*(3), 174–85. https://doi.org/10.1007/s10049-015-0013-0

Rose, N. (2001). The Politics of Life Itself. *Theory Culture Society, 18*(1), 1–30.

Roth, J.A. (1972). Staff and Client Control Strategies in Urban Hospital Emergency Services. *Urban Life and Culture Urban Life and Culture, 1*(1), 39–60.

Röttger, J., Blümel, M., Fuchs, S., and Busse, R. (2014). Assessing the Responsiveness of Chronic Disease Care: Is the World Health Organization's Concept of Health System Responsiveness Applicable? *Social Science & Medicine, 113*, 87–94. https://doi.org/10.1016/j.socscimed.2014.05.009

Ruegenberg, A., Schmiedhofer, M., Kreutzberg, A., Henschke, C., Möckel, M., and Slagman, A. (2024). Blackbox: Psychosoziale Fälle in der Notaufnahme. *Medizinische Klinik – Intensivmedizin und Notfallmedizin, 119*(1), 10–17. https://doi.org/10.1007/s00063-022-00981-x

Savage, M., Cunningham, N., Devine, F., Friedman, S., Laurison, D., McKenzie, L. et al (2015). *Social Class in the 21st Century*. Penguin Random House UK.

Schaeffer, D., and Hämel, K. (2020). Kooperative Versorgungsmodelle. In P. Kriwy and M. Jungbauer-Gans (Eds), *Handbuch Gesundheitssoziologie* (pp 463–80). Springer Fachmedien Wiesbaden. https://doi.org/10.1007/978-3-658-06392-4_26

Schaeffer, D., Berens, E.-M., Gille, S., Griese, L., Klinger, J., de Sombre, S. et al (2021). *Gesundheitskompetenz der Bevölkerung in Deutschland vor und während der Corona Pandemie: Ergebnisse des HLS-GER 2*. https://pub.uni-bielefeld.de/download/2950305/2950403/HLS-GER%202_Ergebnisbericht.pdf

Schaeffer, D., Berens, E.-M., Vogt, D., Gille, S., Griese, L., Klinger, J. et al (2021). Health Literacy in Germany: Findings of a Representative Follow-up Survey. *Deutsches Artzeblatt International, 118*(43), 723–29.

Scherer, M., Lühmann, D., Kazek, A., Hansen, H., and Schäfer, I. (2017). Patients Attending Emergency Departments: A Cross-Sectional Study of Subjectively Perceived Treatment Urgency and Motivation for Attending. *Dtsch Arztebl International, 114*(39), 645–52.

Schilling, H. (2019). *Aller Se Chercher: Urban Youth's Making of Livelihood in Unstable Work in Abidjan and Berlin.* Humboldt-Universität zu Berlin.

Schilling, H. (2023). *Globalized Urban Precarity in Berlin and Abidjan: Young Men and the Digital Economy.* Manchester University Press.

Schinkel, W., and Noordegraaf, M. (2011). Professionalism as Symbolic Capital: Materials for a Bourdieusian Theory of Professionalism. *Comparative Sociology, 10*(1), 67–96. https://doi.org/10.1163/156913310X514083

Schmiedhofer, M., Searle, J., Slagman, A., and Möckel, M. (2017). Inanspruchnahme zentraler Notaufnahmen: Qualitative Erhebung der Motivation von Patientinnen und Patienten mit nichtdringlichem Behandlungsbedarf. *Das Gesundheitswesen, 79*(10), 835–44.

Schmiedhofer, M., Möckel, M., Slagman, A., Frick, J., Ruhla, S., and Searle, J. (2016). Patient Motives Behind Low-Acuity Visits to the Emergency Department in Germany: A Qualitative Study Comparing Urban and Rural Sites. *BMJ Open, 6*(11), e013323. https://doi.org/10.1136/bmjopen-2016-013323

Schubert, L., Naujoks, F., Störmann, P., Rüsseler, M., Herrmann, E., Chobotsky, H. et al (2022). Zwischen Notfall und Fehleinsatz – eine retrospektive Analyse der Einsätze eines Notarzteinsatzfahrzeugs in Frankfurt am Main von 2014 bis 2019. *Notfall + Rettungsmedizin.* https://doi.org/10.1007/s10049-022-01097-7

Schwartz, B. (1975). *Queuing and Waiting: Studies on the Social Organization of Access and Delay.* University of Chicago Press.

Searle, J., Muller, R., Slagman, A., Schäfer, C., Lindner, T., Somasundaram, R. et al (2015). Überfüllung der Notaufnahmen [journal article]. *Notfall + Rettungsmedizin, 18*(4), 306–15. https://doi.org/10.1007/s10049-015-0011-2

Seeger, I. (2019). *Ambulante Notfallversorgung in Deutschland: Verloren zwischen den Sektoren.* Dissertation, Carl von Ossietzky Universität Oldenburg. http://oops.uni-oldenburg.de/4117/1/seeamb19.pdf

Seeger, I., Klausen, A., Thate, S., Flake, F., Peters, O., Rempe, W. et al (2021). Gemeindenotfallsanitäter als innovatives Einsatzmittel in der Notfallversorgung: Erste Ergebnisse einer Beobachtungsstudie. *Notfall + Rettungsmedizin, 24*(3), 194–202. https://doi.org/10.1007/s10049-020-00715-6

Sefrin, P. (2003). Geschichte der Notfallmedizin in Deutschland – unter besonderer Ber ücksichtigung des Notarztdienstes. *An aethesiol Intensivmed Notfallmed Schmerzther, 38*, 623–9.

Sefrin, P. (2024). Referentenentwurf zur Reform der Notfallversorgung. *NOTARZT*, *40*(04), 187–8. https://doi.org/10.1055/a-2349-4411
Sefrin, P. (2025). Rettungsdienst als Teil des Gesetzes zur Notfallversorgung. *NOTARZT*(EFirst). https://doi.org/10.1055/a-2749-5624
Sefrin, P., Händlmeyer, A., and Kast, W. (2015). Leistungen des Notfall-Rettungsdienstes [Performance of the Emergency Service]. *Der Notarzt*, *31*(04), S34–S48. https://doi.org/10.1055/s-0035-1552705
Seim, J. (2017). The Ambulance: Toward a Labor Theory of Poverty Governance. *American Sociological Review*, *82*(3), 451–75. https://doi.org/10.1177/0003122417702367
Seim, J. (2020). *Bandage, Sort, and Hustle: Ambulance Crews on the Front lines of Urban Suffering*. University of California Press.
Seim, J. (2021). Participant Observation, Observant Participation, and Hybrid Ethnography. *Sociological Methods & Research*, *0*(0), 0049124120986209. https://doi.org/10.1177/0049124120986209
Sellin, S.M.E. (2011). *Der Einfluss einer standardisierten Notrufabfrage auf die Struktur des Notrufgesprächs und die Dispositionsqualität bei Fällen von Herz-Kreislauf- Stillstand*. Dissertation, Charité – Universitätsmedizin Berlin. https://refubium.fu-berlin.de/handle/fub188/8341
Shim, J.K. (2010). Cultural Health Capital: A Theoretical Approach to Understanding Health Care Interactions and the Dynamics of Unequal Treatment. *Journal of Health and Social Behavior*, *51*(1), 1–15. https://doi.org/10.1177/0022146509361185
Shim, J.K. (2014). *Heart-Sick: The Politics of Risk, Inequality, and Heart Disease*. New York University Press.
Sieber, F., Kotulla, R., Urban, B., Groß, S., and Prückner, S. (2020). Entwicklung der Frequenz und des Spektrums von Rettungsdiensteinsätzen in Deutschland. *Notfall + Rettungsmedizin*, *23*(7), 490–96. https://doi.org/10.1007/s10049-020-00752-1
Silva, E.B. (2016). Unity and Fragmentation of the Habitus. *The Sociological Review*, *64*(1), 166–83. https://doi.org/10.1111/1467-954X.12346
Slagman, A., Fischer-Rosinský, A., Legg, D., Schmieder, K., and Möckel, M. (2023). Identification of Low-Acuity Attendances in Routine Clinical Information Documented in German Emergency Departments. *BMC Emerg Med*, *23*(1), 64. https://doi.org/10.1186/s12873-023-00838-2
Small, M.L. (2013). Weak Ties and the Core Discussion Network: Why People Regularly Discuss Important Matters with Unimportant Alters. *Social Networks*, *35*(3), 470–83. https://doi.org/10.1016/j.socnet.2013.05.004
Small, M.L. (2017). *Someone to Talk to*. Oxford University Press.
Small, M.L., and McCrory Calarco, J. (2022). *Qualitative Literacy: A Guide to Evaluating Ethnographic and Interview Research*. University of California Press. https://doi.org/10.1525/9780520390676

Small, M.L., and Sukhu, C. (2016). Because They Were There: Access, Deliberation, and the Mobilization of Networks for Support. *Social Networks*, *47*, 73–84. https://doi.org/10.1016/j.socnet.2016.05.002

Smith, D.E. (2005). *Institutional Ethnography: A Sociology for People*. Alta Mira Press.

Smollan, R.K. (2013). Trust in Change Managers: The Role of Affect. *Journal of Organizational Change Management*, *26*(4), 725–47. https://doi.org/10.1108/JOCM-May-2012-0070

Somasundaram, R., Geissler, A., Leidel, B.A., and Wrede, C.E. (2018). Beweggründe für die Inanspruchnahme von Notaufnahmen: Ergebnisse einer Patientenbefragung. *Gesundheitswesen*, *80*(7), 621–7.

Somasundaram, R., Gümbel, D., Poloczek, S., Hasselmann, H., Seybold, J., and Ekkernkamp, A. (2021). *Notfallversorgung in Berlin – heute und morgen: 'It Takes a System to Save a Life'*. https://edoc.bbaw.de/opus4-bbaw/frontdoor/deliver/index/docId/3644/file/BBAW_Denkanstoss8_Somasundaram_et_al.pdf

Soss, J., Fording, R., and Schram, S.F. (2011). The Organization of Discipline: From Performance Management to Perversity and Punishment. *Journal of Public Administration Research and Theory*, *21*, i203–32. https://doi.org/10.1093/jopart/muq095

Spiegel (2017). Mehrheit der Patienten ist kein Notfall. *Spiegel*. https://www.spiegel.de/gesundheit/diagnose/notaufnahme-mehrheit-der-patienten-ist-kein-notfall-a-1177280.html

Spiegel (2018). Überfüllte Rettungsstellen Notfall Notaufnahme. *Spiegel*. https://www.spiegel.de/gesundheit/diagnose/ueberfuellte-notaufnahmen-jeder-sieht-sich-selbst-als-notfall-a-1215087.html

Staab, P., and Vogel, B. (2014). Laufbahn (trajectoire). In G. Fröhlich and B. Rehbein (Eds), *Bourdieu-Handbuch: Leben – Werk – Wirkung* (pp 163–5). J.B. Metzler. https://doi.org/10.1007/978-3-476-01379-8_34

Statista (2020). *Anzahl der Mitglieder und Versicherten der gesetzlichen und privaten Krankenversicherung in den Jahren 2014 bis 2020 (in Millionen)*. https://de.statista.com/statistik/daten/studie/155823/umfrage/gkv-pkv-mitglieder-und-versichertenzahl-im-vergleich/

Statistisches Bundesamt [Destatis] (2024). *12,4 Millionen Behandlungen in Notfallambulanzen im Jahr 2023*. https://www.destatis.de/DE/Presse/Pressemitteilungen/2024/12/PD24_N061_23.html#:~:text=Wie%20das%20Statistische%20Bundesamt%20%28Destatis%29%20mitteilt%2C%20wurden%20in,Wert%20seit%20Beginn%20der%20Erfassung%20im%20Jahr%202018.

Steedman, C. (2000). Enforced Narratives: Stories of Another Self. In T. Cosslett, C. Lury, and P. Summerfield (Eds), *Feminism and Autobiography: Texts, Theories, Methods* (pp 25–39). Routledge.

Steensland, B. (2006). Cultural Categories and the American Welfare State: The Case of Guaranteed Income Policy. *American Journal of Sociology*, *111*(5), 1273–326. https://doi.org/10.1086/499508

Stevenson, F.A., Leydon-Hudson, G., Murray, E., Seguin, M., and Barnes, R. (2021). Patients' Use of the Internet to Negotiate about Treatment. *Social Science & Medicine*, *290*, 114262. https://doi.org/10.1016/j.socscimed.2021.114262

Stivers, T., and McCabe, R. (2021). Dueling in the Clinic: When Patients and Providers Disagree about Healthcare Recommendations. *Social Science & Medicine*, *290*, 114140. https://doi.org/10.1016/j.socscimed.2021.114140

Stivers, T., and Timmermans, S. (2020). Medical Authority under Siege: How Clinicians Transform Patient Resistance into Acceptance. *Journal of Health and Social Behavior*, *61*(1), 60–78. https://doi.org/10.1177/0022146520902740

Strauss, A.L., Fagerhaugh, S., Suczek, B., and Wiener, C. (1982). The Work of Hospitalized Patients. *Social Science & Medicine*, *16*(9), 977–86. https://doi.org/10.1016/0277-9536(82)90366-5

Strazdins, L., Griffin, A.L., Broom, D.H., Banwell, C., Korda, R., Dixon, J., Paolucci, F., and Glover, J. (2011). Time Scarcity: Another Health Inequality? *Environment and Planning A: Economy and Space*, *43*(3), 545–559. https://doi.org/10.1068/a4360

Street, A. (2012). Seen by the State: Bureaucracy, Visibility and Governmentality in a Papua New Guinean Hospital. *TAJA.*, *23*, 1–21.

Struzik, J., Bell, J., Pustułka, P., and Ślusarczyk, M. (2018). Handling Ambivalence: Transnational Health Practices and Migrant Evaluations of Health Services. In M. Ślusarczyk, P. Pustułka, and J. Struzik (Eds), *Contemporary Migrant Families: Actors and Issues* (pp 48–73). Cambridge Scholars Publishing.

Suderland, M. (2014a). Disposition (disposition). In G. Fröhlich and B. Rehbein (Eds), *Bourdieu-Handbuch: Leben – Werk – Wirkung* (pp 73–75). J.B. Metzler. https://doi.org/10.1007/978-3-476-01379-8_15

Suderland, M. (2014b). Hysteresis (hystérésis). In G. Fröhlich and B. Rehbein (Eds), *Bourdieu-Handbuch: Leben – Werk – Wirkung* (pp 127–29). J.B. Metzler. https://doi.org/10.1007/978-3-476-01379-8_26

SVR Gesundheit (2018). *Bedarfsgerechte Steuerung der Gesundheitsversorgung* [Gutachten]. https://www.svr-gesundheit.de/fileadmin/Gutachten/Gutachten_2018/Gutachten_2018.pdf

Threadgold, S. (2018). Bourdieu Is not a Determinist: Illusio, Aspiration, Reflexivity and Affect. In G. Stahl, D. Wallace, C. Burke, and S. Threadgold (Eds), *International Perspectives on Theorizing Aspirations: Applying Bourdieu's Tools* (pp 36–50). Bloomsbury.

Ticktin, M. (2017). A World Without Innocence. *American Ethnologist*, *44*(4), 577–90. https://doi.org/10.1111/amet.12558

Tilly, C. (1998). *Durable Inequality*. University of California Press.

Tilly, C. (2004). Reasons Why. *Sociological Theory*, *22*(3), 445–54. https://doi.org/10.1111/j.0735-2751.2004.00228.x

Tilly, C. (2006). *Why? What Happens When People Give Reasons … and Why*. Princeton University Press.

Tilly, C. (2008). *Credit and Blame*. Princeton University Press. https://doi.org/10.2307/j.ctt7sqfk

Timm, L.H. (2018). *Strukturierte Ersteinschätzung im Rettungsdienst in Anlehnung an das Manchester-Triage-System (MTS)*. Charité – Universitätsmedizin Berlin. https://refubium.fu-berlin.de/bitstream/handle/fub188/3773/Diss_L.H.Timm.pdf;jsessionid=99697BF885B50FB3197A7A1302EFAE19?sequence=1

Timmermans, S. (2020). The Engaged Patient: The Relevance of Patient–Physician Communication for Twenty-First-Century Health. *Journal of Health and Social Behavior*, *61*(3), 259–73. https://doi.org/10.1177/0022146520943514

Timmermans, S., and Epstein, S. (2010). A World of Standards but not a Standard World: Toward a Sociology of Standards and Standardization. *Annual Review of Sociology*, *36*(1), 69–89. https://doi.org/10.1146/annurev.soc.012809.102629

Timmermans, S., and Kolker, E.S. (2004). Evidence-Based Medicine and the Reconfiguration of Medical Knowledge. *Journal of Health and Social Behavior*, *45*, 177–93.

Timmermans, S., and Oh, H. (2010). The Continued Social Transformation of the Medical Profession. *Journal of Health and Social Behavior*, *51*, S94–S106. https://doi.org/10.1177/0022146510383500

Timmermans, S., and Tavory, I. (2012). Theory Construction in Qualitative Research: From Grounded Theory to Abductive Analysis. *Sociological Theory*, *30*(3), 167–86.

Timmons, S., and Nairn, S. (2015). The Development of the Specialism of Emergency Medicine: Media and Cultural Influences. *Health*, *19*(1), 3–16. https://doi.org/10.1177/1363459314530737

Travaglia, J.F., and Braithwaite, J. (2009). Analysing the 'Field' of Patient Safety Employing Bourdieusian Technologies. *Journal of Health Organization and Management*, *23*(6), 597–609. https://doi.org/10.1108/14777260911001626

Tyler, I. (2015). Classificatory Struggles: Class, Culture and Inequality in Neoliberal Times. *The Sociological Review*, *63*(2), 493–511. https://doi.org/10.1111/1467-954x.12296

Uscher-Pines, L., Pines, J., Kellermann, A., Gillen, E., and Mehrotra, A. (2013). Emergency Department Visits for Nonurgent Conditions: Systematic Literature Review. *Am J Manag Care*, *19*(1), 47–59.

Vassy, C. (2001). Categorisation and Micro-Rationing: Access to Care in a French Emergency Department. *Sociology of Health and Illness*, *23*(5), 615–32.

Veenstra, G., and Burnett, P.J. (2014). A Relational Approach to Health Practices: Towards Transcending the Agency-Structure Divide. *Sociology of Health & Illness*, *36*(2), 187–98. https://doi.org/10.1111/1467-9566.12105

Vogel, J.A., Rising, K.L., Jones, J., Bowden, M L., Ginde, A.A., and Havranek, E.P. (2019). Reasons Patients Choose the Emergency Department over Primary Care: A Qualitative Metasynthesis. *Journal of General Internal Medicine*, *34*(11), 2610–19. https://doi.org/10.1007/s11606-019-05128-x

Volker, B. (2020). Social Capital Across the Life Course: Accumulation, Diminution, or Segregation? *Network Science*, *8*(3), 313–32. https://doi.org/10.1017/nws.2020.26

Wacquant, L. (2002). Review Symposium: Scrutinizing the Street: Poverty, Morality, and the Pitfalls of Urban Ethnography. *The American Journal of Sociology.*, *107*(6), 1468.

Wacquant, L. (2005a). Carnal Connections: On Embodiment, Apprenticeship, and Membership [journal article]. *Qualitative Sociology*, *28*(4), 445–74. https://doi.org/10.1007/s11133-005-8367-0

Wacquant, L. (2005b). Shadowboxing with Ethnographic Ghosts: A Rejoinder. *Symbolic Interaction*, *28*(3), 441–7. https://doi.org/10.1525/si.2005.28.3.441

Wacquant, L. (2016). A Concise Genealogy and Anatomy of Habitus. *The Sociological Review*, *64*(1), 64–72. https://doi.org/10.1111/1467-954X.12356

Wahlster, P., Czihal, T., Gibis, B., and Henschke, C. (2020). Sektorenübergreifende Entwicklungen in der Notfallversorgung: Eine Umfassende Analyse Ambulanter und Stationärer Notfälle von 2009 bis 2015 [Developments in Emergency Care – Analysis of Emergency Cases in In- and Outpatient Care from 2009 To 2015 in Germany]. *Gesundheitswesen*(EFirst). https://doi.org/10.1055/a-0820-3904

Wamsiedel, M. (2018). Reasonableness: Legitimate Reasons for Illegitimate Presentations at the ED. *Sociology of Health & Illness*, *40*(8), 1347–60. https://doi.org/10.1111/1467-9566.12776

Wamsiedel, M. (2020). Credibility Work and Moral Evaluation at the ED. *Social Science & Medicine*, *248*, 112845. https://doi.org/10.1016/j.socscimed.2020.112845

Wang, Y. (2016). Homology and Isomorphism: Bourdieu in Conversation with New Institutionalism. *The British Journal of Sociology*, *67*(2), 348–70. https://doi.org/10.1111/1468-4446.12197

Waring, J., Allen, D., Braithwaite, J., and Sandall, J. (2016). Healthcare Quality and Safety: A Review of Policy, Practice and Research. *Sociology of Health & Illness*, *38*(2), 198–215. https://doi.org/10.1111/1467-9566.12391

Watkins-Hayes, C. (2009). *The New Welfare Bureaucrats: Entanglements of Race, Class, and Policy Reform*. University of Chicago Press.

Watkins-Hayes, C. (2019). *Remaking a Life: How Women Living with HIV/AIDS Confront Inequality*. University of California Press.

Wehler, M., Kalch, A., Bilandzic, H., and Händl, T. (2022). Gesundheitskompetenz und Notfallverhalten. *Notfall + Rettungsmedizin*, *25*(6), 427–33. https://doi.org/10.1007/s10049-021-00859-z

Wellman, B., and Wortley, S. (1990). Different Strokes from Different Folks: Community Ties and Social Support. *American Journal of Sociology*, *96*(3), 558–88. https://doi.org/10.1086/229572

Wellman, B., Wong, R.Y.-l., Tindall, D., and Nazer, N. (1997). A Decade of Network Change: Turnover, Persistence and Stability in Personal Communities. *Social Networks*, *19*(1), 27–50. https://doi.org/10.1016/S0378-8733(96)00289-4

Wendt, C. (2003). Vertrauen in Gesundheitssysteme. *Berliner Journal für Soziologie*, *13*(3), 371–393. https://doi.org/10.1007/BF03204675

Wendt, C. (2007). Sinkt das Vertrauen in Gesundheitssysteme? Eine vergleichende Analyse europäischer Länder. *WSI-Mitteilungen*, 7, 380–6. https://doi.org/10.5771/0342-300X-2007-7-380

Wendt, C., and Thompson, T. (2004). Social Austerity versus Structural Reform in European Health Systems: A Four-Country Comparison of Health Reforms. *International Journal of Health Services*, *34*(3), 415–33. https://doi.org/10.2190/dj9q-f2gy-w18r-4c1j

Williams, B., Coyle, J., and Healy, D. (1998). The Meaning of Patient Satisfaction: An Explanation of High Reported Levels. *Soc Sci Med*, *47*(9), 1351–9. https://doi.org/10.1016/s0277-9536(98)00213-5

Willis, K., Collyer, F., Lewis, S., Gabe, J., Flaherty, I., and Calnan, M. (2016). Knowledge Matters: Producing and Using Knowledge to Navigate Healthcare Systems. *Health Sociology Review*, *25*(2), 202–16. https://doi.org/10.1080/14461242.2016.1170624

Wingfield, A.H. (2019). *Flatlining: Race, Work, and Health Care in the New Economy*. University of California Press.

Zelizer, V.A. (2006). Why and How to Read Why?. *Qualitative Sociology*, *29*(4), 531–4. https://doi.org/10.1007/s11133-006-9049-2

Zelizer, V.A. (2012). How I Became a Relational Economic Sociologist and What Does That Mean? *Politics & Society*, *40*(2), 145–74. https://doi.org/10.1177/0032329212441591

Zentralinstitut für die kassenärztliche Versorgung in der Bundesrepublik Deutschland (2022). *SmED – Strukturierte medizinische Ersteinschätzung in Deutschland*. https://www.zi.de/smed

Zussman, R. (2010). Trusting Doctors: The Decline of Moral Authority in American Medicine by Jonathan B. Imber. *American Journal of Sociology*, *115*(4), 1337–8.

Index

References to figures appear in *italic* type; those in **bold** type refer to tables.
References to endnotes show both the page number and the note number (142n1).

S

T